Heart, Brain and Mental Health Disparities for LGBTQ People of Color

"Health psychology is no longer captive to Eurocentric, heteronormative, transphobic assumptions. Psychological scientists and clinicians, proud to serve our racial/ethnic minority and LGBTQ communities, now use powerful theories and methods to advance our communities' health. This visionary volume makes our discoveries more widely known, and frames a bold agenda for the next generation of our work.

In this exemplary book, James J. García brings together gifted established and emerging voices. Grounded in evolutions in the minority stress model, intersectionality, and the science of allostatic load, the contributors here center resilience and strengths-based approaches to improving heart, brain, and mental health among LGBTQ People of Color. With penetrating, critical, synthetic scholarship, the writers in this volume make a convincing case for what works and what remains to be discovered.

Prepare yourself for an encounter with what psychology is becoming and can become, breaking down no-longer-needed clinical, social, and health silos, and divisions between science and practice! For some readers, this book brings together what we've been fighting for all our lives, no longer marginalized in psychology. For others, this volume will disrupt implicit biases and embedded prejudices, false separations among nature, nurture, and social context, and clinical and research methods that, far too often still, do not just exclude but damage LGBTQ People of Color.

Everyone committed to ending health disparities for LGBTQ People of Color will be empowered and excited by this timely and necessary book."
—Richard Ruth, *Associate Professor Emeritus of Clinical Psychology and Founding Core Faculty, LGBT Health Policy and Practice Graduate Certificate Program at The George Washington University, USA*

"This is an original, refreshing and innovative text on health disparities experienced by LGBTQ people of color. It is theoretically wide-ranging, presents current state-of-the-science research focusing on communities of color, and promises to inform research, theory, and practice in the important area of health inequalities. It is an essential text for those of us researching ethnic and sexual disparities in health."
—Rusi Jaspal, *Professor of Psychology at Nottingham Trent University, UK*

James J. García
Editor

Heart, Brain and Mental Health Disparities for LGBTQ People of Color

palgrave
macmillan

Editor
James J. García
Department of Psychology
School of Health and Community Well-Being
University of La Verne
La Verne, CA, USA

ISBN 978-3-030-70059-1   ISBN 978-3-030-70060-7   (eBook)
https://doi.org/10.1007/978-3-030-70060-7

This Palgrave Macmillan imprint is published by the registered company Springer Nature Switzerland AG.
The registered company address is: Gewerbestrasse 11, 6330 Cham, Switzerland

First, this book is devoted to LGBTQ people in history who came before me, namely fierce Trans Women of Color like Marsha P. Johnson, Silvia Rivera, and Miss Major-Griffin Gracy. Their relentless advocacy, coupled with their unapologetic stance as resistance, made it possible for me and others in my communities to have the visibility and freedom to exist in societies today. This text is also dedicated to LGBQ People of Color who want to continue the tremendous work of achieving dignity and respect for our communities. To be honest, this edited collection would not have been possible without the amazing contributions of the book chapter authors, many who identify as racial/ethnic and/or LGBTQ—I am proud to call these fabulous scholars my dear colleagues and friends for life. Lastly, I want to acknowledge and center my immediate family, who continue to learn to embrace me as a Gay Latinx person—though at times difficult, they keep me hopeful that acceptance within my racial/ethnic community as a Gay man is possible. En primer lugar, este libro está dedicado a las personas LGBTQ que me precedieron, a saber, mujeres Trans de Color feroces como Marsha P. Johnson, Silvia Rivera y Miss Major-Griffin Gracy. Su incansable defensa, junto con su postura de resistencia sin complejos, ha hecho posible que yo y otros en mis comunidades tengamos la visibilidad y la libertad de existir en las sociedades de hoy. Este texto también está dedicado a las personas de color LGBQ que desean continuar el tremendo trabajo de lograr la dignidad y el respeto por nuestras comunidades. Para ser honesto, esta colección editada no hubiera sido posible sin las asombrosas contribuciones de los autores de los capítulos del libro, muchos de los cuales se identifican como raciales / étnicos y/o LGBTQ. Me enorgullece llamar a estos fabulosos académicos mis queridos colegas y amigxs de por vida. Por último, quiero reconocer y centrar a mi familia inmediata, que sigue aprendiendo a aceptarme como una persona Gay y Latinx; aunque a veces es difícil, me mantienen con la esperanza de que la aceptación dentro de mi comunidad racial/étnica como hombre Gay es posible.

CONTENTS

Notes on Contributors

Maleeha Abbas, B.Sc. Neuropsychological assessments with people from different racial/ethnic and other minority backgrounds, health disparities between people of color, and dementia.

Benjamin Aguilera, B.S. Advocacy for communities of color and social welfare policy.

Alvin P. Akibar, Ph.D. Sexual minority and gender-diverse people of color health and mental health.

Matthew Alcala, M.A., M.S. LGBTQ populations of color, microaggressions, HIV/AIDS prevention, and substance use disorders.

Aldo Barrita, B.A. Impact of racial, ethnic, and sexual identity microaggressions on marginalized individuals.

Caleb N. Chadwick, Ph.D. Scholarship, teaching, and clinical service specializing within the LGBTQ+ community.

Cirleen DeBlaere, Ph.D. Minority stress and mental health of marginalized populations, resiliency factors, and multicultural competence in therapy. She has served on multiple editorial boards (e.g., *Journal of Counseling Psychology*) and her work has been recognized with multiple national awards (e.g., *Woman of the Year Award; Women of Color Psychologies Award*).

James J. García, Ph.D. Racial/ethnic and LGBTQ cardiovascular/cerebrovascular health and health disparities, namely the role of intersectional discrimination in racial/ethnic LGBTQ health.

Mia Kijak, B.S. Social/personality psychology, specifically in studying the relationship between personality and sexual orientation/gender identity in LGBTQ PoC.

Khashayar F. Langroudi, Psy.D. Intersectionality, gender and sexual minorities, Muslim mental health, eating disorder.

Nadine Nakamura, Ph.D. She is co-chair of the APA LGB Guidelines Revisions Task Force and has recently published a co-edited book *LGBTQ Mental Health: International Perspectives and Experiences.*

Amy Prescott, B.A. Impact of larger LGBTQ community on multiple minorities, including structural determinants that affect the well-being of LGBTQ individuals.

Stephen Ramos, M.A. Behavioral medicine, health behaviors in chronic illness populations, and harm/risk reduction.

Dylan G. Serpas, B.S. Mechanisms by which health disparities arise in marginalized communities and the modifiable risk factors that may reduce the burden of their disproportionate incidence.

Monique J. Williams, MSPA, Ph.D. Identifying health disparities and improving health outcomes among marginalized populations.

David G. Zelaya, Ph.D. Minority stress, intersectionality, and health disparities among individuals with multiple marginalized identities. Clinically, he is interested in cultural competency with Latinx Spanish-speaking populations. He is the recipient of numerous social justice awards and an APA Minority Fellow.

CHAPTER 1

Preface and Introduction: Why Is There a Need for a Book Like This?

James J. García

Abstract As an introductory part, this chapter focuses on the rationale for why there is a need for a text highlighting racial/ethnic LGBTQ PoC heart, brain, and mental health disparities experienced by these communities. In particular, the unique role of intersectional discrimination as a mechanism for these disparities is centered. Terms used throughout the book are defined and the layout/sections of the edited text are explained. Through the unique incorporation of minority stress, intersectionality, and allostatic load frameworks, this timely edited collection presents a holistic and biopsychosocial analysis of LGBTQ PoC well-being, focused on the heart, brain, and psychological health.

Keywords LGBTQ PoC History • Minority Stress • Allostatic Load • Intersectional Discrimination

J. J. García (✉)
Department of Psychology, School of Health and Community Well-Being, University of La Verne, La Verne, CA, USA
e-mail: JGarcia4@laverne.edu

J. J. García (ed.), *Heart, Brain and Mental Health Disparities for LGBTQ People of Color*,
https://doi.org/10.1007/978-3-030-70060-7_1

1

Growing up as a gay Latinx person, I saw very few people like me represented in the media, education, and society at large. Throughout my formative years, my existence as a person of color (PoC) existed along a separate path with my gay identity, which often left me feeling like I was "pulled" to exist either as a gay or Latinx person in different contexts. To no surprise, I felt that I was "too gay" to belong in majority heterosexual Latinx spaces, as I perceived no support—and at times discrimination—for my sexual orientation from these circles. I also was "too brown" to be myself in the predominantly white and racist West Hollywood scene, a large and visible lesbian, gay, bisexual, transgender, and queer (LGBTQ) space in Los Angeles, California. As I expanded my circle of friends and chosen family, many of whom were visible racial/ethnic LGBTQ persons, I began to realized I was not alone: marginalization from racial/ethnic communities and racial/ethnic discrimination within LGBTQ spaces are real and often experienced by LGBTQ PoC, who live, love, and exist at the intersections of their racial/ethnic and LGBTQ identities.

During my graduate training, several experiences demonstrated to me that this social phenomenon was also present in the scientific literature. More specifically, my journey to study Latinx health disparities left me with disappointment, as there was—and continues to be—a lack of representation of Latinx (and other racial/ethnic) LGBTQ communities in research. Fast forward to today, my inspiration for this edited text draws from personal experiences and my professional career. To this end, this edited book is written with the explicit intent of highlighting racial/ethnic LGBTQ PoC heart, brain, and mental health disparities experienced by members of these communities, but also centering the unique role of intersectional discrimination as a mechanism for these disparities.

Paying Homage to Racial/Ethnic LGBTQ Trailblazers

To understand how I came to have the extraordinary opportunity to become the editor of a text like this, we must honor the LGBTQ PoC trailblazers who came before and after the Queer Liberation Movement. Oftentimes, the uprising of 1969 at the Stonewall Inn in New York is credited with the beginnings of the liberation movement for LGBTQ PoC. However, it is important to know that racial/ethnic LGBTQ persons existed well before this uprising, with many fighting and resisting the oppressive powers of heterosexism, homophobia, transphobia, and whiteness prior to this movement (NBC News, 2020; Neta, 2017). Outside the U.S., Amelio Robles, a transgender man of Afro-Mexican descent from the state of Guerrero, México, left his home in 1910 and began living his authentic life as a male. He enlisted to be part of the Mexican Revolutionaries. After the revolution, he applied for government pension for his military service but the Mexican government would only recognize him and his pension through his birth name, which was female. After 20 years of petitioning to the Mexican government, and well into his eighties, Robles was the first Mexican Revolution veteran who was successfully granted recognition by the Mexican government as a male *veterano*. Gladys Bentley, known as "Harlem's most famous Lesbian" in the 1930s during the Harlem Renaissance, performed as an openly gender-bending Black person singing the blues with a top hat and tuxedo. Gonzalo "Tony" Segura was a Cuban-American who founded and led the New York chapter of the Mattachine Society, a large gay rights advocacy group that was based in California—his leadership spread the influence of this gay rights group to the East Coast. José Julio Sarria was born in San Francisco, CA, to Colombian parents and served during World War II. As a drag performer, José was arrested in the early 1960s by police who raided gay bars regularly to arrest "female impersonators" for "crimes." Bayard Rustin, a Black LGBTQ activist, was pivotal in advising Reverend Martin Luther King, Jr., and organizing the 1963 March on Washington. He was arrested in 1953 for having sex with two men in a car in Pasadena, CA—he served 50 days in county jail and had to register as a sex offender. In 2020, Governor Gavin Newsom pardoned Rustin, indicating that he was unjustly punished because of his sexuality and sexual orientation in 1953.

As demonstrated, LGBTQ PoC have resisted the effects of racism and heterosexism, homophobia, and transphobia in society prior to the Stonewall uprising. Nonetheless, the Stonewall resistance had trans PoC who were among the boldest voices in the Queer Liberation Movement. Celebrating her 25th birthday at Stonewall, Marsha P. Johnson, a Black trans woman, was the first to resist. Sylvia Rivera, a Latinx Trans woman, was seen as the first to throw bottles at police officers who raided the Stonewall that night. Also, in attendance was Miss Major Griffin-Gracy, a Black trans woman, and fierce LGBTQ community organizer and advocate. Through their actions, trans women of color (TWoC) have embodied resistance against heterosexism, transphobia, and racism from society; yet, these persons have not received proper credit by their own LGBTQ community for their efforts. Additionally, TWoC are treated by society with violence, as Black and Latinx TWoC experience high rates of physical and sexual assault, often being killed by perpetrators because of their gender identities and/or gender expression. In 2020 alone, 33 TWoC, mostly Black and Latinx, were murdered and their stories are not centered or are often misreported by the police (Human Rights Campaign, 2020). People like Neulisa Luciano Ruiz, from Toa Baja, Puerto Rico, were known for being humble and noble in their community. Monica Diamond who was killed in Charlotte, North Carolina, in March 2020, who was very active in the LGBTQ nightlife, as the co-owner of an event promotion company and co-CEO of the International Mother of the Year Pageantry system, where they honored LGBTQ mothers in the community. The loss of these women impacts not only their immediate loved ones but also the TWoC community at large. Importantly, the disproportionately high murder of TWoC has extended to 2021, which is on track to be a deadlier year (compared to 2020) for Black and Latinx Trans Women. To this end, community-based organizations have become strong supports for TWoC. For example, the TransLatina Coalition of Los Angeles, as a local community-based organization, provides support to trans Latinx and other TWoC, as illustrated with the experiences of Daniela Hernandez, who had gay epithets shouted at her in MacArthur Park in Los Angeles, with perpetrators brutally stabbing her multiple times and slicing her throat (Los Angeles Times, 2020). Luckily, she is alive but this hate crime illustrates how TWoC are treated by society, with their lives seen as dispensable and cut short. Though this is not an exhaustive list of people, these experiences highlight the ongoing history of oppression for LGBTQ PoC before and after Stonewall.

HIGHLIGHTING A NEED

Fast forward to today, LGBTQ PoC are a growing population (Gallup Poll, 2018). However, scarce evidence on the health of LGBTQ PoC exists. In particular, there are limited data on the heart, brain, and mental health for those who identify as racial/ethnic and LGBTQ persons. As such, this edited collection aims to fill this gap, by presenting a critical analysis of current research, as well as highlighting what is not known (but must be known) in the arena of heart, brain, and mental health and health disparities for LGBTQ PoC who live in the U.S.

A Comment on Terminology

As the reader will see, throughout this text there are a variety of terms used by book chapter authors to identify LGBTQ PoC. However, there is a need to comment on why this text is dedicated to the broad umbrella of LGBTQ PoC. Most data to date do not disaggregate LGBTQ findings by race/ethnicity (Barnett et al., 2019), which presents a disservice to the racial/ethnic communities represented in the literature.

To present broad findings for LGBTQ from racial/ethnic communities, many terms used by the contributors of this text illustrate the heterogeneity in identifying these communities. For example, some of the contributors use LGBTQ PoC as a way to refer to these communities as a broad group. Others use the term Sexual and Gender Minorities of Color (SMoC) or Sexual Gender Minority People of Color (SGM PoC). Some use the term racial/ethnic sexual/gender minorities (SGMs) to describe these communities. Moreover, racial/ethnic LGBTQ is also used to denote members of these communities in a broad sense. As it relates to gender identity, the reader will notice the terms gender-diverse PoC, gender-expansive PoC, and gender minorities of color to acknowledge the diversity of gender identities, namely queer, non-conforming, and transgender identities for PoC. The term Transgender and Gender-Non-Conforming (TGNC) PoC is also used to refer to racial/ethnic people who have these diverse gender identities. Therefore, it is important to understand that all of these terms refer to those who identify as LGBTQ and racial/ethnic people broad communities. Though broad terms allow for the organization of findings, this approach does little to disaggregate data by race/ethnicity; this is a critique of the literature published to date. To the extent possible, and if available in cited articles' methodology, the contributors will highlight which racial/ethnic groups are represented in cited studies so that the reader can understand for whom findings are most applicable. Importantly, there are guidelines available from the Williams Institute that help researchers who want to assess sexual orientation/gender identity but do not know how to do this.

Layout of this Text

The following are key questions explored in this edited collection: (1) What trends in heart, brain, and mental health exist for LGBTQ PoC? (2) What health disparities are found in heart, brain, and mental health of LGBTQ PoC? (3) To what extent is the role of intersectional discrimination highlighted or explored in heart, brain, and mental health of LGBTQ

PoC? (4) With a focus toward a strength-based approach, what resilience factors exist among LGBTQ PoC and how can these strengths be fostered to promote thriving/flourishing (not simply surviving) of these communities?

To address these questions, the text is broken down into different parts. The first three chapters focus on theoretical frameworks. For example, the first framework introduced is the minority stress model by Ilan Meyer (2003) to understand the role of minority stress in health disparities, including an identification of risk and resilience factors in the heart, brain, and mental health of LGBTQ PoC. Next, Kimberlé Crenshaw's intersectional framework, drawn from Black feminism and critical race theory, is explicated (Carbado, Crenshaw, Mays, & Tomlinson, 2013). Finally, Bruce McEwan's allostatic load framework, defined as the cumulative effects of adversity that produces a wear and tear of systems involved in heart, brain, and mental health (McEwen, 1998), is discussed in the context of health disparities experienced by LGBTQ PoC. These three introductory chapters provide strong theoretical foundations to describe racial/ethnic LGBTQ heart, brain, and mental health disparities.

The second part, LGBTQ PoC Heart Health, has chapters focusing on the limited, yet mounting, literature regarding bio-behavioral and psychosocial risk factors for cardiovascular diseases (CVDs) in LGBTQ PoC. Given CVDs are the leading cause of death around the world (World Health Organization, 2017), the first chapter draws from the guiding frameworks presented at the beginning of the text to inform CVD risk factor burden in racial/ethnic LGBTQ PoC. In particular, the role of intersectional discrimination is highlighted as a potential mechanism that creates and increases risk of developing CVDs. The second chapter of this section contains a discussion on the relationship of heart health and the Human Immunodeficiency Virus (HIV). For some readers, the inclusion of HIV within a chapter dedicated to CVDs may be somewhat confusing. Yet, given that HIV medications have extended life for people living with HIV (PLWH), comorbidity in diseases of aging are on the rise in PLWH, namely CVDs (Hanna et al., 2016). To this end, this chapter focuses on the comorbidity of HIV and CVDs in LGBTQ PoC, providing evidence that despite being seen as separate disease processes, the literature suggests there may be high comorbidity for racial/ethnic LGBTQ.

The third part, LGBTQ PoC Brain Health, contains a chapter dedicated to presenting the developing literature on stroke risk burden in LGBTQ PoC. Similar to the heart health section, the reader may be confused by the inclusion of HIV in the context of brain health for the second chapter; however, comorbidity of HIV with neurocognitive impairments are common in PLWH (Temereanca et al., 2020), and there may be potentially high impact specifically for LGBTQ PoC. The importance of this chapter emerged from evidence indicating that neurocognitive impairments are seen in PLWH, despite undetectable levels of HIV; therefore, the brain health of PLWH is also reviewed in the context of the "Undetectable = Untransmittable" movement.

Part four, LGBTQ PoC Mental health, contains a chapter centered on the prevalence of mental disorders, and argues for closer attention to the role of intersectional discrimination in substance use and mental health, proposing that adolescence is a critical period for the development of mental health issues for LGBTQ youth of color (Murphy & Hardaway, 2017). Moreover, the second chapter presents psychosocial risk and resilience perspectives for the mental health of LGBTQ PoC, highlighting a need to examine systemic factors and resilience in these communities.

The Conclusions section has chapters focusing on the importance of studying resilience in LGBTQ PoC to understand how these communities exist, survive, and thrive in today's society. Though survival is a minimum, this chapter centers on limited data related to the heterogeneity in operationalizing resiliency as a promotive factor for heart, brain, and mental health for LGBTQ PoC, proposing a call for deliberate action to center LGBTQ PoC persons in future research efforts. Lastly, the second chapter ends with identifying key local, state, and federal policies that hinder heart, brain, mental health thriving of these communities.

SUMMARY

Through the unique incorporation of minority stress, intersectionality, and allostatic load frameworks, this timely edited collection presents a holistic and biopsychosocial analysis of LGBTQ PoC well-being, focused on the heart, brain, and psychological health. Few edited books exist that attempt to do this, as some dedicating no more than four chapters to this endeavor. Overall, this edited collection has the explicit goal of informing research, theory, and practice that influence the lives and well-being of LGBTQ PoC. This text accomplishes this by presenting current state-of-the-science research focused with these communities to continue the work of promoting LGBTQ PoC heart, brain, and psychological health.

REFERENCES

Barnett, A. P., del Río-González, A. M., Parchem, B., Pinho, V., Aguayo-Romero, R., Nakamura, N., ... Zea, M. C. (2019). Content analysis of psychological research with lesbian, gay, bisexual, and transgender people of color in the United States: 1969–2018. *American Psychologist, 74*(8), 898. https://doi.org/10.1037/amp0000562

Carbado, D. W., Crenshaw, K. W., Mays, V. M., & Tomlinson, B. (2013). Intersectionality: Mapping the movements of a theory. *Du Bois review: Social Science Research on Race, 10*(2), 303–312. https://doi.org/10.1017/S1742058X13000349

Gallup. (2018). U.S. estimates of LGBT population rises to 4.5%. https://news.gallup.com/poll/234863/estimate-lgbt-population-rises.aspx

Hanna, D. B., Guo, M., Bůžková, P., Miller, T. L., Post, W. S., Stein, J. H., ... Shikuma, C. M. (2016). HIV infection and carotid artery intima-media thickness: Pooled analyses across 5 cohorts of the NHLBI HIV-CVD collaborative. *Clinical Infectious Diseases, 63*(2), 249–256. https://doi.org/10.1093/cid/ciw261

Human Rights Campaign. (2020). Fatal violence against the transgender and gender non-conforming community in 2020. Retrieved from https://www.hrc.org/resources/violence-against-the-trans-and-gender-non-conforming-community-in-2020.

Los Angeles Times. (2020). Transgender woman "brutally stabbed" at MacArthur park, police say. Retrieved from https://www.latimes.com/california/story/2020-10-06/transgender-woman-brutally-stabbed-downtown-los-angeles.

McEwen, B. S. (1998). Stress, adaptation, and disease: Allostasis and allostatic load. *Annals of the New York Academy of Sciences, 840*(1), 33–44. https://doi.org/10.1111/j.1749-6632.1998.tb09546.x

Meyer, I. H. (2003). Prejudice, social stress, and mental health in lesbian, gay, and bisexual populations: Conceptual issues and research evidence. *Psychological Bulletin, 129*(5), 674–697. https://doi.org/10.1037/0033-2909.129.5.674

Murphy, J., & Hardaway, R. (2017). LGBTQ adolescents of color: Considerations for working with youth and their families. *Journal of Gay and Lesbian Mental Health, 21*(3), 221–227. https://doi.org/10.1080/19359705.2017.1320741

NBC News. (2020). 16 queer black pioneers who made history. Retrieved from https://www.nbcnews.com/feature/nbc-out/black-history-month-17-lgbtq-black-pioneers-who-made-history-n1130856?fbclid=IwAR3GQH7VgvOwswfViQpy9KWOnU1MUUE3S6vWhsMQojHQ92GmxWYdY-WlW5I.

Neta. (2017). 21 LGBTQ Latinx historical figures you should know about. Retrieved from https://netargv.com/2017/10/19/21-lgbtq-latinx-historical-figures-know/?fbclid=IwAR3fxG0ls7Lk7IapkGnpn8U9_CXtxYvEYbiPMbgY1HVqlSFw25MM0AcLMmI.

Temereanca, A., Ene, L., Rosca, A., Diaconu, C. C., Luca, A., Burlacu, R., ... Ruta, S. (2020). Neurocognitive impairment in the combined antiretroviral therapy era in a Romanian cohort of young adults with chronic HIV infection. *AIDS Research and Human Retroviruses, 36*(5), 367–372. https://doi.org/10.1007/s13365-014-0275-1

World Health Organization. (2017). Cardiovascular diseases (CVDs). Retrieved from https://www.who.int/news-room/fact-sheets/detail/cardiovascular-diseases-(cvds).

PART I

Theoretical Frameworks for LGBTQ PoC Heart, Brain and, Mental Health Disparities

CHAPTER 2

Minority Stress in the Study of LGBTQ PoC Health Disparities

Monique J. Williams and Dylan G. Serpas

Abstract To understand LGBTQ PoC health disparities, this chapter centers stress and its insidious effects on the body. Continued exposure to stressful events contributes to serious health issues, including cardiovascular diseases (CVDs), cerebrovascular diseases, and mental health disorders. Stress functions as cumulative vulnerabilities contributing to maintenance of health disparities for racial/ethnic LGBTQ. Although there are various conceptual models to understand the psychosocial, bio-behavioral, and physiological factors pertaining to exposure and reactivity to stress for minoritized groups, this chapter focuses on the widely cited minority stress model of Ilan Meyer as it centers LGBTQ communities. It also

M. J. Williams (✉)
Master of Science in Community Medicine Program, School of Medicine, Keck Graduate Institute, Claremont, CA, USA
e-mail: drmoniquejwilliams@gmail.com

D. G. Serpas
Department of Psychology, California State University, Fullerton, Fullerton, CA, USA

J. J. García (ed.), *Heart, Brain and Mental Health Disparities for LGBTQ People of Color*,
https://doi.org/10.1007/978-3-030-70060-7_2

13

details a theoretical rationale for using Meyer's model as a framework to contextualize the experiences of LGBT PoC as it relates to heart, brain, and mental health.

Keywords Minority Stress Theory • LGBTQ PoC Health • Intersectionality

To help understand LGBTQ PoC health disparities, this chapter will center stress and its insidious effects on the body. To start, stress is the body's natural response to meet the demands of physical, mental, and emotional challenges (National Institutes of Mental Health [NIMH], 2020). Continued exposure to stressful events contributes to serious health issues, including cardiovascular diseases (CVDs), cerebrovascular diseases, and mental health disorders (NIMH, 2020). These stressors function as cumulative vulnerabilities that contribute to the maintenance of health disparities for marginalized groups subjected to additional stressors by virtue of society's response to their identities, including racial/ethnic LGBTQ. Although there are various conceptual models to understand the psychosocial, bio-behavioral, and physiological factors pertaining to exposure and reactivity to stress for minoritized groups, including the cumulative vulnerability minority stress model of Hector Myers (Myers, Lewis, & Parker-Dominguez, 2003), this chapter will focus on the widely cited minority stress model of Ilan Meyer (2003), as it centers LGBTQ communities.

The social experiences of minoritized people in society have drawn the attention of researchers. Indeed, separate lines of research suggest stress reactions and negative physiological and psychological health outcomes are increased for LGBTQ (Caceres et al., 2017; Sutter & Perrin, 2016) and racial/ethnic communities or people of color (PoC; Benjamin et al., 2019; Williams & Mohammed, 2009). However, LGBTQ PoC face different, yet related, stigma, prejudice, and discrimination from society at large (i.e., heterosexism within their racial/ethnic communities) and broader LGBTQ communities, resulting in additional within-group social marginalization (Meyer, 2010). Thus, this chapter will detail a theoretical rationale for using Meyer's (2003) model as a framework to contextualize the experiences of LGBT PoC as it relates to heart, brain, and mental health.

Theoretical Rationale of the Minority Stress Model

Broadly speaking, minority stress is one extensively documented psychosocial mechanism that contributes and maintains health disparities for socially minoritized communities. Indeed, racial/ethnic minorities and sexual/gender minorities (SGMs) experience a disproportionate incidence and magnitude of discrimination related to society's minoritization of their identities. As a result, this discrimination—as a psychosocial stressor—represents a unique pathway in the risk and development of negative health outcomes for socially marginalized groups.

One widely cited theory, the Minority Stress Theory (MST) developed by Ilan Meyer (1995), defines minority stress as excess social stress experienced by members of historically marginalized groups. Importantly, holding minoritized identities, in and of itself, is not stressful; rather, it is society's response to these that perpetuates stigma and creates stressful experiences for people who hold these minoritized identities This model captures the ways in which various factors, including proximal and distal stressors, function as cumulative vulnerabilities contributing to negative health outcomes, either directly or indirectly (Meyer, 2003). Proximal minority stressors refer to internal perceptions and responses to negative external experiences based on self-stigmas such as internalized homophobia (Meyer, 2003). Distal minority stressors include external stressors brought about by society such as harassment and/or discrimination (e.g., microaggressions) in schools, workplaces, housing, and health-care environments (Ramirez & Paz Galupo, 2019). These hostile and stressful social experiences are associated with greater prevalence of depression, anxiety, substance use disorders, suicide (Lee, Gamarel, Bryant, Zaller, & Operario, 2016; Plöderl & Tremblay, 2015), chronic health conditions, obesity, and overall poor physical health in SGMs compared to heterosexual counterparts (Gonzales & Henning-Smith, 2017). These findings are not isolated to just the U.S.—an international study of 86,000 SGMs across 28 European countries revealed that in countries with higher levels of SGM societal prejudice and stigma, lower quality of life was reported by SGM persons (Pachankis & Bränström, 2018).

Minority Stress and Health

Given that the psychosocial experiences described earlier are stressful for SGMs, it is reasonable to extend Meyer's model for the study of health outcomes among LGBTQ PoC. In fact, many studies support this conjecture. Exposure to racial/ethnic discrimination directly influence physiological systems, thereby increasing risk for poor physical and mental health outcomes, including CVDs, obesity, smoking, alcohol consumption, anxiety, depression, and greater inflammatory biomarkers linked to chronic diseases in domestic and international studies (Benjamin et al., 2019; Ferdinand, Paradies, & Kelaher, 2015; Gil-González et al., 2014; Harris, Stanley, & Cormack, 2018; Panza et al., 2019). Therefore, racial/ethnic discrimination is considered a unique psychosocial stressor (Brondolo, Brady, Libby, & Pencille, 2011), with meta-analytic and systematic review evidence indicating the negative impact of this stressor on mental and physical health, either directly or indirectly, as a social determinant of health (Paradies et al., 2015).

A closer examination of Meyer's (2003) minority stress model proposes that distal and proximal processes are the mechanisms by which SGMs attain negative health outcomes. Given the explicit focus on SGMs, this framework outlines a minority stress process that we argue can be adapted to also include the unique effects of racial/ethnic discrimination experienced by racial/ethnic SGMs. By considering racial/ethnic and sexual orientation/gender identity–based discrimination as unique sources of minority stress, this intersectional approach contributes to broader and more comprehensive assessments of mechanisms involved in the development of LGBTQ PoC health disparities. Thus, we suggest extending the MST model to examine psychosocial stressors experienced by LGBTQ PoC, much like Cyrus (2017) and Whitfield, Walls, Langenderfer-Magruder, and Clark (2014) argued, as this offers a more inclusive representation of the intersectional lived experiences (not just identifying as two identities) of racial/ethnic LGBTQ.

Intersectionality

Despite our reasonable assertion, the intersectional health literature remains fragmented, as separate bodies of literature document these unique and adverse experiences faced by both SGMs and PoC. However, it is sensible to expect that existence as a racial/ethnic LGBTQ person in society is associated with unique psychosocial stressors, which then are associated with greater psychosocial stress, thereby increasing the risk for negative health outcomes. Indeed, recent studies support this conjecture with the use of intersectionality theory. For example, Veenstra (2011) provided broad evidence on the utility of intersectionality theory to understand the interaction between race, gender, social class, and sexual orientation on health. Experiencing multiple sources of discrimination, compared to simply just one source, is associated with poorer mental and physical health in U.S.-based and international LGBTQ samples (Cormack, Stanley, & Harris, 2018; Ramirez & Paz Galupo, 2019). Similar findings are echoed across a variety of disciplines including sociology, psychology, psychiatry, and medicine (Grollman, 2014; Remedios & Snyder, 2018; Vargas, Huey Jr., & Miranda, 2020).

Though research on LGBTQ PoC health is emerging, minimal empirical investigations focus on the impact of intersectional stressors on health. Justifiably, this research is critical, as LGBTQ PoC experience distinct forms of intersectional stress and discrimination related to lived experiences at the intersection of multiple socially minoritized identities (Balsam, Molina, Beadnell, Simoni, & Walters, 2011; Sutter & Perrin, 2016). Of the limited literature, one study found that LGB Black and Latinx demonstrated higher rates of substance abuse compared to heterosexual same race/ethnicity counterparts (Mereish & Bradford, 2014). Additionally, Cerezo and Ramirez (2020) found that among lesbian, queer, and bisexual Latinx and Blacks, racial/ethnic and sexual orientation-based discrimination uniquely predicted alcohol-related outcomes. Moreover, English, Rendina, and Parsons (2018) found that among Black, Latinx, and multiracial gay and bisexual men, intersectional discrimination was associated with higher levels of emotion regulation problems, anxiety, and depression symptoms. Importantly, excess psychosocial stress can be harmful to one's health, which may result in double or even triple jeopardy (i.e., experiencing additional stress for each added layer of minoritized identity beyond what is experienced by members of single minority groups) among LGBTQ PoC (Meyer, 2010). For example, Ramirez and Paz Galupo (2019) explored the effects of distal (i.e., LGBT PoC microaggressions and daily heterosexism/racism) and proximal (i.e., internalized stigma, identity salience, and sexual orientation rumination) stressors on mental health in majority Black, Latinx, and Asian American LGB. Findings revealed that, when combined, distal and proximal stressors held more predictive power of mental health than when examined independently (Ramirez & Paz Galupo, 2019). Despite the harmful effects of adverse experiences related to intersectional identities, those who hold minoritized identities demonstrate remarkable strength and resilience, a testament to their ability to exist in the face of social adversity, as described later in this edited collection.

Not a New Framework, But One That Is Vital

Implementation of an intersectional perspective in the context of LGBTQ PoC health status is not new. In fact, this perspective was noted by the Institute of Medicine (IOM, 2011), which recognized there are communities within SGMs based on demographic characteristics such as race/ethnicity, age, socioeconomic positions, and education, which influence each community's experiential reality and health. This perspective has been highlighted by work from the American Psychological Association (APA, 2012), which recommended mental health professionals working with SGMs consider that individuals who are SGM PoC must navigate complex social environments as intersectional beings (APA, 2012).

Given the unique psychosocial experiences faced by LGBTQ PoC, it is vital to use an intersectional perspective to adequately capture the experiential realities of these communities (Cole, 2009). Living at the intersection of multiple socially marginalized identities is accompanied by adverse psychological, social, and emotional experiences secondary to systemic and historical prejudice, bias, and discrimination in society. Therefore, integrating Meyer's (2003) framework, in addition to an intersectionality perspective, is key to contextualizing these experiences for LGBTQ PoC to avoid intersectional invisibility in the literature (Ramirez, Gonzalez, & Paz Galupo, 2018).

INTERSECTIONAL STRESSORS EXPERIENCED BY LGBTQ PoC

The diversity of LGBTQ PoC communities warrants an examination of the unique impact that psychosocial experiences have on these socially minoritized communities (Cyrus, 2017). This is important so that researchers and practitioners effectively intervene and reduce negative health outcomes associated with multiple minority stressors (Cyrus, 2017). Regrettably, removal and exclusion of SGMs in national aging and disability surveys by the Trump Administration enforces additional barriers to examining LGBTQ health, particularly for those who self-identify as LGBTQ PoC (Cahill & Makadon, 2017). Moreover, studies often group lesbian women with gay men and label samples as LGBTQ. Such practices are inherently flawed, as they place limitations on accurately counting SGMs and gloss over adverse intersectional experiences (Nadal, Whitman, Davis, Erazo, & Davidoff, 2016). Additionally, while categorizing diverse groups into a general LGBTQ population may be convenient in exploratory research, results and implications neglect the needs of certain segments of communities, most notably Trans Women of Color (TWoC; Nadal et al., 2016). Such a focus is important, as qualitative data indicate Latinx Trans women report negative health-care experiences (e.g., discrimination from providers), which impacts their willingness to seek care (Abreu et al., 2020; Howard et al., 2019). This is important, as there is small but growing literature in the U.S. on trans Latinx and other TWoC in health care, with racism as an explanatory variable at the forefront and center of the science. Taken together, research on the distinct experiences of LGBTQ PoC warrants additional empirical attention to address each community's distinct unmet needs.

The social experiences that LGBTQ PoC face negatively impact these communities and may lead to concealment of their identities (Dyar, Feinstein, Eaton, & London, 2018) and increased maladaptive coping (Gaylord-Harden & Cunningham, 2009). The intersectional discrimination of SGM and racial/ethnic minority identity is also demonstrated in other ways, including anti-LGBTQ discrimination within racial/ethnic group, racial/ethnic discrimination within the LGBTQ community from majority white and other PoC SGM groups (Ramirez & Paz Galupo, 2019). To illustrate this, Szymanski and Sung (2010) found heterosexism in communities of color, racial/ethnic discrimination among LGBTQ persons, and internalized heterosexism-predicted psychological stress in Asian American LGB. Notably, the study sample was majority LGB (96%), only 4% transgender, predominantly Chinese (28%) and Filipino (19%), and sexual orientation was collapsed into one monolithic group for analysis. As the LGBTQ PoC population grows and diversifies, increased acceptance, support, and efforts to identify health disparities must be included as well as interventions to confront unmet health needs of LGBTQ PoC (Cyrus, 2017).

Psychosocial Factors in Health Disparities for LGBTQ PoC

The immediate environments that people are exposed to impact their ability to successfully navigate the world. Indeed, these experiences influence how people's bodies respond to psychosocial stressors, with direct influence on the autonomic nervous system, all of which are inextricably related to the heart, brain, and emotions (Bennett, Rohleder, & Sturmberg, 2018). SGM PoC are at greater risk of exposure to experiences of intersectional discrimination due to chronic societal marginalization (Balsam et al., 2011). Chronic activation of physiological systems, resulting from experiences of intersectional discrimination, including elevated and sustained release of damaging inflammatory proteins, hormones, and increased blood pressure and heart rate, produce adverse physical and mental health, as attempts to self-regulate via homeostasis is not achieved (Bennett et al., 2018).

More importantly, the impact of intersectional discrimination on the heart, brain, and mental health of LGBTQ communities is frequently cited, yet rarely tested. For example, in research in CVD prevalence among Black lesbian and bisexual women, controlling for modifiable risk factors (e.g., smoking, obesity), Black LGB men and Latinx persons who indicated an unsure sexual orientation had a greater CVD burden than heterosexual white counterparts (Caceres et al., 2020); however, intersectional discrimination was not directly tested. As indicated by Parra and Hastings (2018), adverse effects of intersectional discrimination produce physiological stress responses and effect neurobiological regulation, which contribute to greater allostatic load; this is discussed later in this edited text. Nonetheless, there are few studies focused on the impact of intersectional discrimination on physical health (Parra & Hastings, 2018).

As previously identified, LGBTQ PoC are at increased risk for poor mental health outcomes, including depression, anxiety, and psychological well-being (Ramirez & Paz Galupo, 2019). These findings are likely attributable to sustained physiological arousal that LGBTQ PoC naturally respond to as a result of the inherently stressful experiences of living in racist and anti-LGBTQ contexts (Ramirez & Paz Galupo, 2019). Moreover, this sustained activation is adverse, resulting in worse mental health due to cumulative psychosocial battle fatigue, given that these stressors are cumulative in nature and occur across the life span (Ramirez & Paz Galupo, 2019).

Summary

It is critical to focus on the unique heart, brain, and the mental health needs of SGM PoC to increase our understanding of factors impacting this segment of the population and to inform effective interventions. Centering the unique health needs of LGBTQ PoC is important and must be done, particularly by health-care professionals from all disciplines, as there is a necessity to improve the biopsychosocial health of racial/ethnic LGBTQ communities (Bennett et al., 2018).

References

Abreu, R. L., Gonzalez, K. A., Mosley, D. V., Pulice-Farrow, L., Adam, A., & Duberli, F. (2020). 'They feel empowered to discriminate against las chicas:' Latina transgender women's experiences navigating the healthcare system. *International Journal of Transgender Health*. https://doi.org/10.108 0/26895269.2020.1767752

American Psychological Association (APA). (2012). Guidelines for psychological practice with lesbian, gay, and bisexual clients. *American Psychologist, 67*(1), 10–42. https://doi.org/10.1037/a0024659

Balsam, K. F., Molina, Y., Beadnell, B., Simoni, J., & Walters, K. (2011). Measuring multiple minority stress: The LGBT People of Color Microaggressions Scale. *Cultural Diversity and Ethnic Minority Psychology, 17*(2), 163. https://doi.org/10.1037/a0023244

Benjamin, E. J., Muntner, P., Alonso, A., Bittencourt, M. S., Callaway, C. W., Carson, A. P., ... American Heart Association Council on Epidemiology and Prevention Statistics Committee and Stroke Statistics Subcommittee. (2019). Heart disease and stroke statistics-2019 update: A report from the American Heart Association. *Circulation, 139*(10), e56–e528. https://doi.org/10.1161/CIR.0000000000000659

Bennett, J. M., Rohleder, N., & Sturmberg, J. P. (2018). Biopsychosocial approach to understanding resilience: Stress habituation and where to intervene. *Journal of Evaluation in Clinical Practice, 24*(6), 1339–1346. https://doi.org/10.1111/jep.13052

Brondolo, E., Brady, N., Libby, D., & Pencille, M. (2011). Racism as a psychosocial stressor. In R. J. Contrada & A. Baum (Eds.), *Handbook of stress science: Biology, psychology, and health* (pp. 167–184). New York, NY: Springer Publishing Company.

Caceres, B. A., Ancheta, A. J., Dorsen, C., Newlin-Lew, K., Edmondson, D., & Hughes, T. L. (2020). A population-based study of the intersection of sexual identity and race/ethnicity on physiological risk factors for CVD among U.S. adults (ages 18–59). *Ethnicity & Health*, 1–22. https://doi.org/10.108 0/13557858.2020.1740174

Caceres, B. A., Brody, A., Luscombe, R. E., Primiano, J. E., Marusca, P., Sitts, E. M., & Chyun, D. (2017). A systematic review of cardiovascular disease in sexual minorities. *American Journal of Public Health, 107*(4) https://doi.org/10.2105/AJPH.2016.303630

Cahill, S. R., & Makadon, H. J. (2017). If they don't count us, we don't count: Trump administration rolls back sexual orientation and gender identity data collection. *LGBT Health, 4*(3), 171–173. https://doi.org/10.1089/lgbt.2017.0073

Cerezo, A., & Ramirez, A. (2020). Perceived discrimination, alcohol use disorder and alcohol-related problems in sexual minority women of color. *Journal of Social Service Research*, 1–14. https://doi.org/10.1080/0148837 6.2019.1710657

Cole, E. R. (2009). Intersectionality and research in psychology. *American Psychologist*, *64*(3), 170–180. https://doi.org/10.1037/a0014564

Cormack, D., Stanley, J., & Harris, R. (2018). Multiple forms of discrimination and relationships with health and wellbeing: Findings from national cross-sectional surveys in Aotearoa/New Zealand. *International Journal for Equity in Health*, *17*(26), 1–15. https://doi.org/10.1186/s12939-018-0735-y

Cyrus, K. (2017). Multiple minorities as multiply marginalized: Applying the minority stress theory to LGBTQ people of color. *Journal of Gay & Lesbian Mental Health*, *21*(3), 194–202. https://doi.org/10.1080/1935970 5.2017.1320739

Dyar, C., Feinstein, B., Eaton, N., & London, B. (2018). The mediating roles of rejection sensitivity and proximal stress in the association between discrimination and internalizing symptoms among sexual minority women. *Archives of Sexual Behavior*, *47*(1), 205–218. https://doi.org/10.1007/ s10508-016-0869-1

English, D., Rendina, H. J., & Parsons, J. T. (2018). The effects of intersecting stigma: A longitudinal examination of minority stress, mental health, and substance use among Black, Latino, and multiracial gay and bisexual men. *Psychology of Violence*, *8*(6), 669–679. https://doi.org/10.1037/vio0000218

Ferdinand, A. S., Paradies, Y., & Kelaher, M. (2015). Mental health impacts of racial discrimination in Australian culturally and linguistically diverse communities: A cross-sectional survey. *BMC Public Health*, *15*(1), 401. https://doi.org/10.1186/s12889-015-1661-1

Gaylord-Harden, N. K., & Cunningham, J. A. (2009). The impact of racial discrimination and coping strategies on internalizing symptoms in African American youth. *Journal of Youth and Adolescence*, *38*(4), 532–543. https:// doi.org/10.1007/s10964-008-9377-5

Gil-González, D., Vives-Cases, C., Borrell, C., Agudelo-Suárez, A. A., Davó-Blanes, M. C., Miralles, J., & Álvarez-Dardet, C. (2014). Racism, other discriminations and effects on health. *Journal of Immigrant and Minority Health*, *16*(2), 301–309. https://doi.org/10.1007/s10903-012-9743-y

Gonzales, G., & Henning-Smith, C. (2017). Health disparities by sexual orientation: Results and implications from the Behavioral Risk Factor Surveillance System. *Journal of Community Health*, *42*(6), 1163–1172. https://doi.org/10.1007/s10900-017-0366-z

Grollman, E. A. (2014). Multiple disadvantaged statuses and health: The role of multiple forms of discrimination. *Journal of Health and Social Behavior*, *55*(1), 3–19. https://doi.org/10.1177/0022146514521215

Harris, R. B., Stanley, J., & Cormack, D. M. (2018). Racism and health in New Zealand: Prevalence over time and associations between recent experience of racism and health and wellbeing measures using national survey data. *PloS One, 13*(5), e0196476. https://doi.org/10.1371/journal.%20pone.0196476

Howard, S. D., Lee, K. L., Nathan, A. G., Wenger, H. C., Chin, M. H., & Cook, S. C. (2019). Healthcare experiences of transgender people of color. *Journal of General Internal Medicine, 34*(10), 2068–2074. https://doi.org/10.1007/s11606-019-05179-0

Institute of Medicine (IOM). (2011). *The health of lesbian, gay, bisexual, and transgender people: Building a foundation for better understanding.* The National Academies Press.

Lee, J. H., Gamarel, K. E., Bryant, K. J., Zaller, N. D., & Operario, D. (2016). Discrimination, mental health, and substance use disorders among sexual minority populations. *LGBT Health, 3*(4), 258–265. https://doi.org/10.1089/lgbt.2015.0135

Mereish, E. H., & Bradford, J. B. (2014). Intersecting identities and substance use problems: Sexual orientation, gender, race. *and lifetime substance use problems. Journal of Studies on Alcohol and Drugs, 75*(1), 179–188. https://doi.org/10.15288/jsad.2014.75.179

Meyer, I. H. (1995). Minority stress and mental health in gay men. *Journal of Health and Social Behavior, 36*(1), 38–56. http://www.jstor.org/stable/2137286

Meyer, I. H. (2003). Prejudice, social stress, and mental health in lesbian, gay, and bisexual populations: Conceptual issues and research evidence. *Psychological Bulletin, 129*(5), 674–697. https://doi.org/10.1037/0033-2909.129.5.674

Meyer, I. H. (2010). Identity, stress, and resilience in lesbians, gay men, and bisexuals of color. *The Counseling Psychologist, 38*(3), 442–454. https://doi.org/10.1177/0011000009351601

Myers, H. F., Lewis, T. T., & Parker-Dominguez, T. (2003). *Stress, coping, and minority health: Biopsychosocial perspective on ethnic health disparities.* In G. Bernal, J. E. Trimble, A. K. Burlew, & F. T. L. Leong (Eds.), *Handbook of racial & ethnic minority psychology* (pp. 377–400). SAGE Publications Inc.. https://doi.org/10.4135/9781412976008.n19

Nadal, K. L., Whitman, C. N., Davis, L. S., Erazo, T., & Davidoff, K. C. (2016). Microaggressions toward lesbian, gay, bisexual, transgender, queer, and genderqueer people: A review of the literature. *Journal of Sex Research, 53*(4–5), 488–508. https://doi.org/10.1080/00224499.2016.1142495

National Institute of Mental Health (NIMH). (2020). *5 things you should know about stress.* Retrieved from https://www.nimh.nih.gov/health/publications/stress/index.shtml.

Pachankis, J. E., & Bränström, R. (2018). Hidden from happiness: Structural stigma, sexual orientation concealment, and life satisfaction across 28 countries.

Journal of Consulting and Clinical Psychology, 86(5), 403–415. https://doi. org/10.1037/ccp0000299

Panza, G. A., Puhl, R. M., Taylor, B. A., Zaleski, A. L., Livingston, J., & Pescatello, L. S. (2019). Links between discrimination and cardiovascular health among socially stigmatized groups: A systematic review. *PloS One, 14*(6), e0217623. https://doi.org/10.1371/journal.pone.0217623

Paradies, Y., Ben, J., Denson, N., Elias, A., Priest, N., Pieterse, A., ... Gee, G. (2015). Racism as a determinant of health: A systematic review and meta-analysis. *PloS One, 10*(9) https://doi.org/10.1371/journal.pone.0138511

Parra, L. A., & Hastings, P. D. (2018). Integrating the neurobiology of minority stress with an intersectionality framework for LGBTQ-Latinx populations. *New Directions for Child and Adolescent Development, 161*, 91–108. https://doi. org/10.1002/cad.20244. https://doi.org/10.1002/cad.20244

Plöderl, M., & Tremblay, P. (2015). Mental health of sexual minorities: A systematic review. *International Review of Psychiatry, 27*(5), 367–385. https://doi. org/10.3109/09540261.2015.1083949

Ramirez, J. L., Gonzalez, K. A., & Paz Galupo, M. P. (2018). Invisible during my own crisis': Responses of LGBT people of color to the Orlando shooting. *Journal of Homosexuality, 65*(5), 579–599. https://doi.org/10.108 0/00918369.2017.1328217

Ramirez, J. L., & Paz Galupo, M. (2019). Multiple minority stress: The role of proximal and distal stress on mental health outcomes among lesbian, gay, and bisexual people of color. *Journal of Gay & Lesbian Mental Health, 23*(2), 145–167. https://doi.org/10.1080/19359705.2019.1568946

Remedios, J. D., & Snyder, S. H. (2018). Intersectional oppression: Multiple stigmatized identities and perceptions of invisibility, discrimination, and stereotyping. *Journal of Social Issues, 74*(2), 265–281. https://doi.org/10.1111/ josi.12268

Sutter, M., & Perrin, P. B. (2016). Discrimination, mental health, and suicidal ideation among LGBTQ people of color. *Journal of Counseling Psychology, 63*(1), 98–105. https://doi.org/10.1037/cou0000126

Szymanski, D. M., & Sung, M. R. (2010). Minority stress and psychological distress among Asian American sexual minority persons. *The Counseling Psychologist, 38*(6), 848–872. https://doi.org/10.1177/0011000010366167

Vargas, S. M., Huey, S. J., Jr., & Miranda, J. (2020). A critical review of current evidence on multiple types of discrimination and mental health. *American Journal of Orthopsychiatry, 90*(3), 374–390. https://doi.org/10.1037/ ort0000441

Veenstra, G. (2011). Race, gender, class, and sexual orientation: Intersecting axes of inequality and self-rated health in Canada. *International Journal for Equity in Health, 10*(1), 3–11. https://doi.org/10.1186/1475-9276-10-3

Whitfield, D. L., Walls, N. E., Langenderfer-Magruder, L., & Clark, B. (2014). Queer is the new black? Not so much: Racial disparities in anti-LGBTQ discrimination. *Journal of Gay & Lesbian Social Services, 26*(4), 426–440. https://doi.org/10.1080/10538720.2014.955556

Williams, D. R., & Mohammed, S. A. (2009). Discrimination and racial disparities in health: Evidence and needed research. *Journal of Behavioral Medicine, 32*, 20–47. https://doi.org/10.1007/s10865-008-9185-0

CHAPTER 3

Intersectionality, Lived Social Realities, and LGBTQ PoC Health

Alvin P. Akibar and Khashayar F. Langroudi

Abstract A focus on the intersectional experiences of racial/ethnic LGBTQ is important. A large body of research indicates individuals with sexual minority or gender-diverse identities have an increased risk for psychological distress compared to heterosexual counterparts. Despite an increasing focus on sexual and gender minority stress and its implications for mental health, much of this work does not address the minority stress experience associated with the social marginalization of racial/ethnic LGBTQ identities. This chapter focuses on presenting the concept of intersectionality and the real-world impact of living life at the intersections of identities for racial/ethnic LGBTQ.

Keywords Intersectionality • Group Identity • LGBTQ PoC Health

A. P. Akibar (✉)
Department of Psychology, St. Catherine University, St. Paul, MN, USA
e-mail: apakibar162@stkate.edu

K. F. Langroudi
University of San Francisco, San Francisco, CA, USA

© The Author(s), under exclusive license to Springer Nature Switzerland AG 2021
J. J. García (ed.), *Heart, Brain and Mental Health Disparities for LGBTQ People of Color*,
https://doi.org/10.1007/978-3-030-70060-7_3

27

As illustrated in the previous chapter, a focus on the intersectional experiences for racial/ethnic LGBTQ is important. A large body of research indicates individuals with sexual minority (e.g., lesbian, gay, bisexual [LGB]) or gender-diverse identities (e.g., Queer, Transgender, Gender-Non-Conforming [QTGNC]) are at increased risk for psychological distress compared to heterosexual counterparts (Meyer, 1995; 2003). Despite an increasing focus on sexual and gender minority (SGM) stress and its implications for mental health (Meyer, 2003), much of this work does not address the minority stress experience associated with the social marginalization of racial/ethnic LGBTQ identities. This is disheartening, as the literature severely underrepresents sexual and gender minority persons of color (SGMoC), despite the very real impacts of both SGM and race-related stress on mental well-being (Huang et al., 2010), with little visibility of QTGNC people in the scientific literature.

This point is highlighted in several content analyses of literature on sexual minorities of color. For example, Huang et al. (2010) found that research with racial/ethnic and sexual orientation/and gender-diverse persons, while on the increase, has historically been limited. More recently, Barnett et al. (2019) extended this work, finding that despite substantial increases in representation of sexual minorities of color within the literature, transgender People of Color (PoC) are still only nominally represented over the span of a decade since the previous content analysis was conducted. Studies examining links between LGBTQ identities and mental health largely represent experiences of white LGBTQ individuals (Barnett et al., 2019). Further, of the studies of SGM stress that include PoC, most fail to report participants' racial/ethnic identities altogether (Coulter et al., 2014). Likewise, studies that examine issues of racial/ethnic group identity and mental health frequently rely on predominantly cisgender, heterosexual samples (Nadal et al., 2014), or fail to report sexual orientation of participants (Huynh et al., 2014). This leaves SGMoC at the crossroads of inadequate representation in the health literature. Therefore, it is important to critically analyze contributions of racial/ethnic and sexual identities simultaneously, as these uniquely exist at the intersection of these identities (Bowleg, 2008; 2013).

INTERSECTIONALITY

The term *intersectionality* emerged from sociological discussions rooted in intersections of feminist and anti-racist social movements in the 1960s–1970s (hooks, 1984). Kimberlé W. Crenshaw is credited as the first to publish about intersectionality by name, highlighting how multiple reinforcing structures of oppression must be considered together to properly analyze these oppressive societal forces (Carbado, Crenshaw, Mays, & Tomlinson, 2013). Crenshaw's conceptualization initially described the ways Black women were doubly excluded from discourse surrounding feminism in favor of white women, and within anti-racist discussions in favor of Black men. A key principle of intersectionality is that social identities are interdependent and multidimensional. Another crucial tenet of intersectionality is that the intersections of social identities, in combination with experiences at individual level and broader societal context, interact to create distinct social milieus for socially marginalized people, namely LGBTQ PoC.

Perspectives on Intersecting Identities

Much work conceptualizing the intersections of racial/ethnic and SGM identity highlights the mechanisms by which these identities are distinct from one another, and how these differences frame the social experiences for SGMoC. Whereas individuals might avoid discrimination by concealing these identities, it is less likely that these individuals can avoid marginalization based upon their visible and perceived racial/ethnic backgrounds (Choi, Han, Paul, & Ayala, 2011). In his classic work on stigma, Goffman (2009) theorized that individuals with a concealable stigmatized identity face a range of negative consequences if that identity is revealed, which could understandably heighten motivations to conceal it. Once a concealable stigmatized identity is revealed within a social interaction, Goffman argued, an individual may subsequently feel pressure to mitigate negative impressions surrounding their identity. Feelings of stigmatization may prompt individuals to engage in a variety of protective behaviors, ranging from avoidance of the non-stigmatized majority to attempts to pass as members of the majority. Though these strategies may aid in avoiding stigmatization of concealable identities, they negatively impact the mental and physical well-being of those with socially stigmatized identities, particularly LGBTQ PoC (Meyer, 2003).

The unique realities of social inequity for those with both concealable and non-concealable stigmatized identities often leave researchers at a loss for how to adequately measure these intersecting identities. For instance, while some may conceptualize identity intersections as additive forces in the lives of individuals with multiple minority statuses, this approach does accurately depict the experiences of SGMoC (Velez, Watson, Cox Jr., & Flores, 2017). Weber and Parra-Medina (2003) describe the conundrum associated with asking a person who may be oppressed on multiple fronts (for instance, a non-conforming Latinx individual from a low SES background) to identify a single root of that oppression, for which responses can range from messy to uninformative. This challenge is salient in some studies; for example, Díaz, Ayala, Bein, Henne, and Marin (2001) extensively integrate economic factors of homophobia and racism in contextualizing gay and bisexual Latino men's mental health. They acknowledge how stigmatization can both result in, and be exacerbated by, contextual factors such as poverty, through social alienation and isolation from effective coping and treatment resources. To this end, Bowleg (2013) aptly describes this phenomena utilizing a vivid metaphor of a cake: once mixed and baked, the cake cannot simply be reduced to the sum of its individual components. Rather, it is these components, the processes involved in combining them, and the conditions in which they intersect, that determine the final creation (i.e., lived experiences of intersectional beings). Therefore, the totality of intersectional experience (rather than additive or multiplicative perspectives) provides tremendous insight into the realities faced by people who exist at the intersections of their socially minoritized identities (Fattoracci et al., 2020). Other perspectives regarding intersectionality focus on the psychosocial stressor of intersectional discrimination using intracategorical (i.e., unique to particular identity intersections) and intercategorical (i.e., comparative across various intersections) frameworks. As an example, Scheim and Bauer (2019), in their scale validation of the Intersectional Discrimination Index, extend Weber and Parra-Medina's (2003) methodological critique of intersectional research, and propose a framework for intercategorical discrimination research that allows participants to report their experiences with attention paid to the difficulty associated with determining a root cause for their experiences of discrimination.

Intersectional Discrimination and Health

Societal attitudes that disparage identities can be internalized by people, leading to increased harassment and violence against those perceived as part of stigmatized minority groups (Federal Bureau of Investigation, 2016). More specifically, SGMoC navigate a cultural landscape that is discriminatory due to multiple aspects of their identities. In addition to facing multiple potential sources of harassment and discrimination, these experiences of discrimination are further compounded by contexts. For instance, racism within the LGBTQ community may push a Muslim SGMoC refugee in the European Union further from would-be primary sources of support, given potential for familial rejection due to sexual orientation/gender identity. This within-group discrimination is also evidenced across various racial/ethnic groups, such that SGMoC experience heterosexist discrimination within their own cultural groups and families (Malebranche et al., 2009; Siegel & Epstien 1996). This type of harassment by those considered to be part of a person's in-group and broader community contextualizes findings suggesting that SGMoC are less likely to feel supported by the LGBTQ community, compared to White LGBTQ counterparts, or to even consider themselves part of the LGBTQ community.

Beyond the immediate harm caused by experiences of harassment and assault, fear of such harassment can add the burden of stress, further victimizing those already vulnerable to the ire of a cisgender, heterosexual, and white society. For instance, McCabe and colleagues (2010) found that stress linked to experiences of discrimination related to race/ethnicity, gender, and sexuality was associated with increased risk (threefold) for substance use problems. Notably, while this work examined self-reported past-year discrimination based on a limited assessment of race/ethnicity, sexual identity, and gender as separate, SGMoC groups were not disaggregated, and instances of discrimination due to multiple identities simultaneously were not measured. Furthermore, compounding the negative effects of both stigma and psychological difficulty (Hughes & Eliason, 2002), sexual minorities who face psychological difficulties are less likely to seek help for these problems (McCabe et al., 2013). This reduction in help-seeking may be rooted in both the feared and lived experiences of discrimination from healthcare professionals (Beehler, 2001).

GROUP IDENTITY AND RESILIENCE

Research examining psychological outcomes among SMoC is intertwined with the nature of intersecting identities and their associations with mental health outcomes. Findings typical for marginalized groups suggest heightened risk associated with the compounding of stress linked to experiences of homophobia, racism, and less access to mental health resources for SGMoC (Frost & Meyer, 2012). For SGMs, community identification holds mixed implications for well-being, with evidence of both protective and risk factors across outcomes such as substance use, sexual risk behaviors, and mental health (Lelutiu-Weinberger et al., 2013). Rather than a simple multiplicative increase in risk due to the experience of multiple sources of discrimination, these experiences can shape how a person learns to cope with future events (Meyer, 2010). Further, Meyer (2010) suggests that if SGMoC experience successful coping with racial/ethnic discrimination prior to coming out, this buffers the impacts of LGBTQ-related discrimination. This finding is not new, as several studies emphasize that living as a person who holds multiple minority statuses may confer resilience by buffering the negative impact of stigma (e.g., Adams, Cahill, & Ackerlind, 2005; Moradi et al., 2010). Moreover, Frost and Meyer (2012) argue that those who hold multiply disadvantaged minority identities may feel more connected to these identities/cultures than more privileged peers.

Group Identity

A growing body of research examines how individuals' perceptions of their own identities impact their ability to cope with stigmatizing experiences and overall well-being. Moreover, evidence suggests that the strength of identification may substantially frame experiences of SGMoC, to the extent that decisions to be "out" with their LGBTQ identity are framed by intersections of family/community with racial/ethnic, sexual, and gender identities collectively, rather than separately, and not by an individualistic need to be out (Bowleg, Burkholder, Teti, & Craig, 2008).

Indeed, for SGMs, involvement within a broader community may promote feelings of belonging and fulfillment (McMillan & Chavis, 1986; Stone, Nimmons, Salcido Jr., & Schnarrs, 2020), informational support (Rhodes et al., 2015), and lower feelings of anxiety and stress (Woodford, Kulick, & Atteberry, 2015). In their recent work on the ways transgender and non-conforming people find and benefit from community, Stone et al. (2020) found that while these community connections can be useful for coping with traumatic experiences of marginalization, Black and American Indian participants struggled the most in finding in-person LGBTQ community connections, facing difficulties with full inclusion within these communities. They highlight that the pitfalls in identity mismatch of transgender and non-conforming PoC and the broader LGB community groups increase mental health issues, even among particularly resilient TGNC individuals.

Findings often indicate that a stronger sense of commitment to a racial/ethnic group is associated with better mental health outcomes (Rivas-Drake et al., 2014), higher self-esteem (Phinney et al., 2001), and lower anxiety and depressive symptoms (Costigan et al., 2010). However, SGMoC may face racial/ethnic stigmatization within SGM communities and contend with homophobia, biphobia, and transphobia within racial/ethnic communities, namely their proximal families of origin (Bieschke, Paul, & Blasko, 2007). Racist attitudes also persist within LGBTQ spaces under the guise that those who experience sexual orientation or gender identity discrimination cannot be bigoted themselves, or the "just a preference" statements in the context of sexual racism; that is, dating or sexual selection of partners based on race/ethnicity (Balsam, Molina, Beadnell, Simoni, & Walters, 2011). Thus, LGBTQ PoC often struggle to fit in as racial/ethnic and sexual/gender-diverse beings between and within these respective communities.

Identity Conflict

Given the potential for stigmatization within SGM communities of racial/ethnic LGBTQ, balancing the influence of these identities may create a source of unique stress for SGMoC that is not present for White SGM (Sarno, Mohr, Jackson, & Fassinger, 2015). Further evidence indicates protective factors present for heterosexual PoC may not necessarily be generalized to SGMoC. For instance, the influence of positive sexual identity development among SGMoC may be less protective than that of racial/ethnic identity for Black gay and bisexual men (Walker, Longmire-Avital, & Golub, 2015). Similarly, a study of LGBTQ youth of color by Kuper, Coleman, and Mustanski (2014) found that while coping-based racial/ethnic socialization messages can serve as a source of reassurance in the face of discrimination [among 246 participants from Black/

African-American (66.2%), multiracial (14.1%), Hispanic/Latino (13.1%), Native American (0.8%), and other (4.2%) racial/ethnic backgrounds], those who have concerns of parental rejection related to an LGBTQ identity may not necessarily reap the benefits of coping through racial/ethnic socialization messages. Correspondingly, the well-being of SGMoC may not be as strongly and positively related to affiliation as compared to broader White SGM communities. To support this, an exploration of conflicts-in-allegiances (CIA), a person's feelings of perceived incompatibility between racial/ethnic and sexual minority identity, by Sarno et al. (2015) found that 124 LGB participants (representing Asian, Black, Latina/Latino, Native American, Middle Eastern, and multiracial (35.5%) racial/ethnic backgrounds) who identified strongly with both their ethnicity and their sexual orientation experienced less conflict than those who identified with one more strongly than the other. This evidence supports the notion that increased conflict between the predominant salience of either their racial/ethnic or sexual minority identity is associated with increased psychological distress (Santos & VanDaalen, 2016), though this conflict is an all too familiar feeling for many SGMoC (Balsam et al., 2011).

DISCUSSION

In this chapter, we examined literature that addresses intersections of racial/ethnic and SGM identities. The literature suggests a few key topics of concern. Namely, the idea that living with multiple minority statuses exacerbates risk for negative outcomes for SGMoC is rooted in multiple layers of complexity and it is naïve to reduce these lived experiences to parts of a whole for LGBT PoC.

At an individual level, SGMoC may feel conflict between racial/ethnic and sexual identities. Interpersonally, feared or experienced rejection of one or more identity statuses among peers and loved ones may contribute to feelings of isolation. Being perceived as a member of both racial/ethnic and sexual minority groups may identify SGMoC as targets for harassment and discrimination from society, with immediate dangers to physical safety and negative psychological and physical health consequences that are chronic in nature. Given this unique reality for many SGMs, it is important that research continue to emphasize the importance of contexts.

Shifting focus this way can begin to address the overrepresentation of the experiences of White LGB in SGM research (Barnett et al., 2019), as many issues affecting SGM are amplified in impact for PoC (Bridge et al., 2015). Understanding the intersections of these identities can only be done with more attention to how identities interact systemically and individually. The especially complex nature of identity intersections leaves many PoC, and those who occupy multiple socially marginalized identities, wanting representation and basic support from others (Balsam et al., 2011). Concerns of SGMoC are often left unaddressed within research, and much of this deficit may relate to the way researchers conceptualize topics of research, that is, frameworks are predominantly capturing white LGBTQ experiences. Contrary to commonly adopted models of sexual identity development, several studies indicate that SGMoC may face a different set of markers associated with positive identity development, which subsequently impacts their psychological and physical well-being. Therefore, continued research should seek to identify potential sources of resilience at the root of these trends.

CONCLUSIONS

To truly center the experiences of PoC in predominantly scholarly work would require a drastic overhaul of the current norms within the psychological and biomedical literature. The body of research concerning intersectionality, mental health, and physical health has grown substantially in recent years. This increased attention has shed light on several identity-related and intersectional factors that impact mental and physical health outcomes for SGMoC. Though daunting, continued work that examines and remains focused on the experiences of SGMoC is needed to examine ways that these identity-related and intersectional constructs come together to inform health for SGM PoC.

REFERENCES

Adams, E. M., Cahill, B. J., & Ackerlind, S. J. (2005). A qualitative study of Latino lesbian and gay youths' experiences with discrimination and the career development process. *Journal of Vocational Behavior, 66*(2), 199–218. https://doi.org/10.1016/j.jvb.2004.11.002

Balsam, K. F., Molina, Y., Beadnell, B., Simoni, J., & Walters, K. (2011). Measuring multiple minority stress: The LGBT People of Color Microaggressions Scale.

Cultural Diversity and Ethnic Minority Psychology, 17(2), 163–174. https:// doi.org/10.1037/a0023244

Barnett, A. P., del Río-González, A. M., Parchem, B., Pinho, V., Aguayo-Romero, R., Nakamura, N., ..., & Zea, M. C. (2019). Content analysis of psychological research with lesbian, gay, bisexual, and transgender people of color in the United States: 1969–2018. *American Psychologist, 74*(8), 898. https://doi. org/10.1037/amp0000562.

Beehler, G. P. (2001). Original Research: Confronting the culture of medicine: Gay men's experiences with primary care physicians. *Journal of the Gay and Lesbian Medical Association, 5*(4), 135–141. https://doi.org/10.1023/ A:1014210027301

Bieschke, K. J., Paul, P. L., & Blasko, K. A. (2007). Review of empirical research focused on the experience of lesbian, gay, and bisexual clients in counseling and psychotherapy. In K. J. Bieschke, R. M. Perez, & K. A. DeBord (Eds.), *Handbook of counseling and psychotherapy with lesbian, gay, bisexual, and transgender clients* (2nd ed., pp. 293–315). Washington, DC: American Psychological Association. https://doi.org/10.1037/11482-012

Bowleg, L. (2008). When Black + lesbian + woman ≠ Black lesbian woman: The methodological challenges of qualitative and quantitative intersectionality research. *Sex Roles: A Journal of Research, 59*(5–6), 312–325. https://doi. org/10.1007/s11199-008-9400-z

Bowleg, L. (2013). "Once you've blended the cake, you can't take the parts back to the main ingredients:" Black gay and bisexual men's descriptions and experiences of intersectionality. *Sex Roles, 68*(11–12), 754–767. https://doi. org/10.1007/s11199-012-0152-4

Bowleg, L., Burkholder, G., Teti, M., & Craig, M. L. (2008). The complexities of outness: Psychosocial predictors of coming out to others among Black lesbian and bisexual women. *Journal of LGBT Health Research, 4*(4), 153–166. https://doi.org/10.1080/15574090903167422

Bridge, J. A., Asti, L., Horowitz, L. M., Greenhouse, J. B., Fontanella, C. A., Sheftall, A. H., ... Campo, J. V. (2015). Suicide trends among elementary school–aged children in the United States from 1993 to 2012. *JAMA pediatrics, 169*(7), 673–677. https://doi.org/10.1001/jamapediatrics.2015.0465

Carbado, D. W., Crenshaw, K. W., Mays, V. M., & Tomlinson, B. (2013). Intersectionality: Mapping the movements of a theory. *Du Bois Review: Social Science Research on Race, 10*(2), 303–312. https://doi.org/10.1017/ S1742058X13000349

Costigan, C. L., Koryzma, C. M., Hua, J. M., & Chance, L. J. (2010). Ethnic identity, achievement, and psychological adjustment: Examining risk and resilience among youth from immigrant Chinese families in Canada. *Cultural diversity and ethnic minority psychology, 16*(2), 264.

Choi, K. H., Han, C. S., Paul, J., & Ayala, G. (2011). Strategies for managing racism and homophobia among US ethnic and racial minority men who have sex with men. *AIDS Education and Prevention, 23*(2), 145–158. https://doi.org/10.1521/aeap.2011.23.2.145

Coulter, R. W., Kenst, K. S., Bowen, D. J., & Scout. (2014). Research funded by the National Institutes of Health on the health of lesbian, gay, bisexual, and transgender populations. *American Journal of Public Health, 104*(2), e105–e112. https://doi.org/10.2105/AJPH.2013.301501

Díaz, R. M., Ayala, G., Bein, E., Henne, J., & Marin, B. V. (2001). The impact of homophobia, poverty, and racism on the mental health of gay and bisexual Latino men: Findings from 3 U.S. cities. *American Journal of Public Health, 91*(6), 927–932. https://doi.org/10.2105/ajph.91.6.927

Fattoracci, E. S., Revels-Macalinao, M., & Huynh, Q. L. (2020). Greater than the sum of racism and heterosexism: Intersectional microaggressions toward racial/ethnic and sexual minority group members. *Cultural diversity and ethnic minority psychology.*

Federal Bureau of Investigation (2020). *Hate Crime Statistics 2019.* Washington, D.C., U.S. Department of Justice. Retrieved from https://ucr.fbi.gov/hate-crime/2019

Frost, D. M., & Meyer, I. H. (2012). Measuring community connectedness among diverse sexual minority populations. *Journal of Sex Research, 49*(1), 36–49. https://doi.org/10.1080/00224499.2011.565427

Goffman, E. (2009). *Stigma: Notes on the management of spoiled identity.* Simon and Schuster. https://doi.org/10.4324/9780203793343-4.

hooks, B. (1984). *Feminist theory: From margin to center.* Boston, MA: South End.

Huang, Y.-P., Brewster, M. E., Moradi, B., Goodman, M. B., Wiseman, M. C., & Martin, A. (2010). Content analysis of literature about LGB people of color: 1998–2007. *The Counseling Psychologist, 38*(3), 363–396. https://doi.org/10.1177/0011000009335555

Hughes, T. L., & Eliason, M. (2002). Substance use and abuse in lesbian, gay, bisexual and transgender populations. *The Journal of Primary Prevention, 22*(3), 263–298. https://doi.org/10.1023/A:1013669705086

Huynh, Q. L., Devos, T., & Goldberg, R. (2014). The role of ethnic and national identifications in perceived discrimination for Asian Americans: Toward a better understanding of the buffering effect of group identifications on psychological distress. *Asian American journal of psychology, 5*(3), 161.

Kuper, L. E., Coleman, B. R., & Mustanski, B. S. (2014). Coping with LGBT and racial–ethnic-related stressors: A mixed-methods study of LGBT youth of color. *Journal of Research on Adolescence, 24*(4), 703–719. https://doi.org/10.1111/jora.12079

Lelutiu-Weinberger, C., Pachankis, J. E., Golub, S. A., Ja'Nina, J. W., Bamonte, A. J., & Parsons, J. T. (2013). Age cohort differences in the effects of gay-related stigma, anxiety and identification with the gay community on sexual risk and substance use. *AIDS and Behavior,* *17*(1), 340–349. https://doi. org/10.1007/s10461-011-0070-4

Malebranche, D. J., Fields, E. L., Bryant, L. O., & Harper, S. R. (2009). Masculine socialization and sexual risk behaviors among Black men who have sex with men: A qualitative exploration. *Men and masculinities,* 12(1), 90–112.

McMillan, D. W., & Chavis, D. M. (1986). Sense of community: A definition and theory. *Journal of Community Psychology,* *14*(1), 6–23. https://doi.org/1 0.1002/1520-6629(198601)14:1<6::AID-JCOP2290140103>3.0.CO;2-I

McCabe, S. E., Bostwick, W. B., Hughes, T. L., West, B. T., & Boyd, C. J. (2010). The relationship between discrimination and substance use disorders among lesbian, gay, and bisexual adults in the United States. *American Journal of Public Health,* 100(10), 1946–1952.

McCabe, S. E., West, B. T., Hughes, T. L., & Boyd, C. J. (2013). Sexual orientation and substance abuse treatment utilization in the United States: Results from a national survey. *Journal of substance abuse treatment,* 44(1), 4–12.

Meyer, I. H. (1995). Minority stress and mental health in gay men. *Journal of Health and Social Behavior,* *36*(1), 38–56. https://doi.org/10.2307/2137286

Meyer, I. H. (2003). Prejudice, social stress, and mental health in lesbian, gay, and bisexual populations: Conceptual issues and research evidence. *Psychological Bulletin,* *129*(5), 674–697. https://doi.org/10.1037/0033-2909.129.5.674

Meyer, I. H. (2010). Identity, stress, and resilience in lesbians, gay men, and bisexuals of color. *The Counseling Psychologist,* 38(3), 442–454.

Moradi, B., Wiseman, M. C., DeBlaere, C., Goodman, M. B., Sarkees, A., Brewster, M. E., & Huang, Y. P. (2010). LGB of color and white individuals' perceptions of heterosexist stigma, internalized homophobia, and outness: Comparisons of levels and links. *The Counseling Psychologist,* 38(3), 397–424. https://doi.org/10.1177/0011000009335263

Nadal, K. L., Griffin, K. E., Wong, Y., Hamit, S., & Rasmus, M. (2014). The impact of racial microaggressions on mental health: Counseling implications for clients of color. *Journal of Counseling & Development,* 92(1), 57–66.

Phinney, J. S., Horenczyk, G., Liebkind, K., & Vedder, P. (2001). Ethnic identity, immigration, and well-being: An interactional perspective. *Journal of social issues,* 57(3), 493–510.

Rhodes, S. D., Alonzo, J., Mann, L., M. Simán, F., Garcia, M., Abraham, C., & Sun, C. J. (2015). Using photovoice, Latina transgender women identify priorities in a new immigrant-destination state. *International Journal of Transgenderism,* *16*(2), 80–96. https://doi.org/10.1080/1553273 9.2015.1075928.

Rivas-Drake, D., Seaton, E. K., Markstrom, C., Quintana, S., Syed, M., Lee, R. M., ..., & Ethnic and Racial Identity in the 21st Century Study Group. (2014). Ethnic and racial identity in adolescence: Implications for psychosocial, academic, and health outcomes. *Child Development, 85*(1), 40–57. https://doi.org/10.1111/cdev.12200.

Sarno, E. L., Mohr, J. J., Jackson, S. D., & Fassinger, R. E. (2015). When identities collide: Conflicts in allegiances among LGB people of color. *Cultural Diversity and Ethnic Minority Psychology, 21*(4), 550–559. https://doi.org/10.1037/cdp0000026

Santos, C. E., & VanDaalen, R. A. (2016). The associations of sexual and ethnic–racial identity commitment, conflicts in allegiances, and mental health among lesbian, gay, and bisexual racial and ethnic minority adults. *Journal of Counseling Psychology, 63*(6), 668–676. https://doi.org/10.1037/cou0000170

Scheim, A. I., & Bauer, G. R. (2019). The Intersectional Discrimination Index: Development and validation of measures of self-reported enacted and anticipated discrimination for intercategorical analysis. *Social Science & Medicine, 226*, 225–235.

Siegel, K., & Epstein, J. A. (1996). Ethnic-racial differences in psychological stress related to gay lifestyle among HIV-positive men. *Psychological Reports, 79*(1), 303–312.

Stone, A. L., Nimmons, E. A., Salcido, R., Jr., & Schnarrs, P. W. (2020). Multiplicity, race, and resilience: Transgender and non-binary people building community. *Sociological Inquiry, 90*(2), 226–248. https://doi.org/10.1111/soin.12341

Velez, B. L., Watson, L. B., Cox, R., Jr., & Flores, M. J. (2017). Minority stress and racial or ethnic minority status: A test of the greater risk perspective. *Psychology of Sexual Orientation and Gender Diversity, 4*(3), 257. https://doi.org/10.1037/sgd0000226

Walker, J. J., Longmire-Avital, B., & Golub, S. (2015). Racial and sexual identities as potential buffers to risky sexual behavior for Black gay and bisexual emerging adult men. *Health Psychology, 34*(8), 841–846. https://doi.org/10.1037/hea0000187

Weber, L., & Parra-Medina, D. (2003). Intersectionality and women's health: Charting a path to eliminating health disparities. *Advances in Gender Research, 7*, 181–230. https://doi.org/10.1016/s1529-2126(03)07006-1

Woodford, M. R., Kulick, A., & Atteberry, B. (2015). Protective factors, campus climate, and health outcomes among sexual minority college students. *Journal of Diversity in Higher Education, 8*(2), 73–87. https://doi.org/10.1037/a003855

CHAPTER 4

Allostatic Load and the Wear and Tear of the Body for LGBTQ PoC

Dylan G. Serpas and James J. García

Abstract To examine the physiological impact of intersectional discrimination for LGBTQ PoC, this chapter introduces the allostatic load framework to allow for such conceptualization. Indeed, substantial evidence supports a relationship between chronic stress exposure and negative health outcomes. Socially marginalized groups within the U.S. experience unique psychosocial stressors that pose serious psychological and physiological health risks. Using the minority stress framework, and specifying the importance of intersectionality, this chapter also details the available literature on the cumulative effects of marginalization on physiological functioning for LGBTQ PoC, by highlighting the limited literature on health outcomes linked to intersectional discrimination. Thus, this chapter

D. G. Serpas (✉)
Department of Psychology, California State University, Fullerton, Fullerton, CA, USA

J. J. García
Department of Psychology, School of Health and Community Well-Being, University of La Verne, La Verne, CA, USA
e-mail: JGarcia4@laverne.edu

J. J. García (ed.), *Heart, Brain and Mental Health Disparities for LGBTQ People of Color*,
https://doi.org/10.1007/978-3-030-70060-7_4

41

focuses on using the AL model to conceptualize the cumulative impact of marginalization and discrimination for LGBTQ PoC.

Keywords Allostatic Load • Social Marginalization • Intersectional Discrimination

To examine the physiological impact of intersectional discrimination for LGBTQ PoC, this chapter introduces the allostatic load framework to allow for such conceptualization. Indeed, substantial evidence supports a relationship between chronic stress exposure and negative health outcomes (McEwen, 1998; McEwen & Gianaros, 2010; McEwen & Stellar, 1993). Socially marginalized groups within the U.S. experience unique psychosocial stressors that pose serious psychological and physiological health risks. One framework that captures these unique experiences is the Minority Stress Theory (MST), which details psychosocial, bio-behavioral, and physiological factors related to stress (Meyer, 2003), including experiences of discrimination salient to minority social status. This theory identifies proximal (i.e., subjective; e.g., self-stigmatization) and distal (i.e., objective e.g., direct experiences of discrimination) stressors that impact health (Meyer, 2003).

Exposure to marginalization as stress activates autonomic physiological response systems, namely the hypothalamic–pituitary–adrenal (HPA) axis, which secretes hormones used to return the body to equilibrium or homeostasis (McEwen, 1998). This physiological response is referred to as allostasis, or the typical physiological adaptation to stress, promoting survival by protecting the body from damage (Sterling & Eyer, 1988). However, if allostasis is sustained over time, allostatic load (AL) can result. In such instances, damaging alterations in physiological mechanisms occur and contribute to the development of chronic health conditions (e.g., heart diseases, stroke). Using the minority stress framework, and specifying the importance of intersectionality, this chapter details the available literature on the cumulative effects of marginalization on physiological functioning for LGBTQ people of color (PoC), by highlighting the limited literature on health outcomes linked to intersectional discrimination. Thus, the chapter focuses on using the AL model to conceptualize the cumulative impact of marginalization and discrimination for LGBTQ PoC.

ALLOSTATIC LOAD THEORY

The AL framework captures overall system dysregulation or physiological wear and tear on the body due to sustained arousal or stress. This paradigm describes the AL process as a feedback loop that, with repeated activation, triggers in response to chronic stress; overtime, this physically breaks down interdependent bodily systems that are important to individual and social adaptation (McEwen, 1998). Indeed, during times of stress, the body typically engages in a process by which it responds to immediate threats, or acute stressors, to regain homeostasis, a process referred to as allostasis (Sterling & Eyer, 1988). Accordingly, allostasis is the body's innate adaptation to acute stress consisting of stress hormone secretion, which functions to regain homeostasis following the resolved threat.

Stress hormones have protective and harmful effects on the body. These hormones are secreted by multiple systems within the body; however, the body's primary stress response and regulation system is the HPA (Juster, McEwen, & Lupien, 2010). Although stress hormones are vital to stress reactivity and play a role in regaining homeostatic equilibrium, they are also taxing to the body's physiological response systems. That is, if the body's natural stress response system goes unchecked, this can compromise physiological functioning through repeated activation across time. Moreover, when stress hormones continually circulate throughout the body, they interfere with the gene transcription process and decrease the number of neuroreceptors in the brain (McEwen, 1998). This is harmful, as an insufficient number of receptors for stress hormones become available for binding, which inhibits signal transmission to cease the typical stress response. Consequently, a negative feedback loop cannot occur, resulting in a prolonged and sustained stress response (McEwen, 1998). Researchers have examined the AL framework within and outside of the U.S., in countries including Germany, Australia, Finland, Sweden, Scotland, Norway, Finland, and China (see Juster et al., 2010 for a review). As such, the AL framework is widely accepted as a comprehensive model with promising international generalizability in capturing the cumulative effects of chronic stress on the body.

Typically, AL is quantified by using physiological indicators of pathophysiological damage or biological dysfunction. These physiological indicators are referred to as biomarkers and are used to assess the functioning of different physiological systems. Indicators can be divided into those that originate from the HPA axis or non-HPA axis. HPA indicators include cortisol, alpha amylase, interleukin-6 (IL-6), glycosylated hemoglobin (HbA1c), tumor necrosis factor (TNF-a), C-reactive protein (CRP), blood glucose, blood pressure (BP), and cholesterol (i.e., LDL, HDL, total cholesterol), whereas non-HPA axis AL indicators are albumin, creatinine, BMI, and waist-to-hip ratio (Juster et al., 2010). Thus, these biomarkers serve to approximate HPA functioning and will be highlighted throughout this chapter.

SOCIAL ADVERSITY AND THE STRESS RESPONSE

Social adversity is one example of chronic stress that impacts AL burden. More specifically, systematic review evidence indicates that historically marginalized groups, such as PoC, demonstrate greater AL (Beckie, 2012). This robust finding suggests that the social milieu for those from socially minoritized communities is deleterious to health due to societal stigma and discrimination experienced in the form of psychosocial stress. Likewise, it is plausible that these findings may extend to sexual/gender minorities (SGMs) who are PoC, as these communities experience heterosexism, biphobia, transphobia, homophobia, and racism, which negatively impact psychological well-being (Rhodes et al., 2020). Indeed, social experiences that are discriminatory in nature function as chronic and cumulative stressors, disrupting the ability of socially minoritized identities to maintain psychosocial and physiological equilibrium (Parra & Hastings, 2018).

As previously described, AL results from a stress response activated by psychosocial experiences that are cognitively appraised as threats (McEwen, 2000). Correspondingly, the physiological stress system responds as though facing a threat, even if the individual is no longer in the physical vicinity of the stressor. In fact, psychosocial stressors, like discrimination, are linked to physiological stress and inflammatory responses in separate samples of PoC and SGMs (Lucas et al., 2017; Saban et al., 2018). For example, one experimental study has documented nonsignificant trends for increased BP and electrical heart functioning in response to racial/ethnic microaggressions (i.e., subtle discrimination) among Latinx (García, Serpas, & Torres, 2020). Another experimental study reported significant cardiovascular reactivity in the face of anticipated and blatant racial/ethnic discrimination among Latinx (Sawyer, Major, Casad, Townsend, & Mendes, 2012). Moreover, Huynh, Huynh, and Stein (2017) found greater total cortisol output in response to indirect ethnic discrimination among Latinx. In a study with SGMs, Juster and colleagues (2019) observed higher BP among gay and bisexual men compared to hetero-sexual counterparts in a laboratory stress task. Finally, studies conducted outside of the U.S. document higher physiological reactivity among SGMs uniquely linked to SGM-based discrimination (Jacobson, Cohen, & Diamond, 2016; Juster et al., 2015). Thus, considerable evidence supports the notion that social marginalization is a unique psychosocial pathway that increases stress physiological reactivity for PoC and LGBTQ people.

Allostatic Load in PoC

Social marginalization and stigma related to a person's race/ethnicity is psychologically stressful and harmful to physical health. Indeed, adverse physiological health consequences from chronic stress disproportionately affect PoC (compared to their white counterparts). Multiple theoretical frameworks describe this phenomenon. For example, James, Hartnett, and Kalsbeek's (1983) seminal work on the concept of *John Henryism* describes the process of detrimental physiological costs from expending high levels of psychological and physiological resources in the face of pro-longed stress exposure, such as when facing chronic instances of racism and discrimination for Black communities. Moreover, Geronimus' (1992) *weathering hypothesis* states that collective chronic stress exposure wears off on the body and leads to accelerated physiological aging or "weathering." Additionally, Clark, Anderson, Clark, and Williams (1999) developed a biopsychosocial model of stress to explain how exposure to racism involves the interplay between multiple environmental and individual-level factors that combine to produce negative health outcomes for PoC. Lastly, Myers, Lewis, and Parker-Dominguez (2003) combined elements from previous stress models to develop a cumulative framework that details the chronic nature of minority stress and AL, with social factors as a central compo-nent in this model. Though tremendous work has gone into developing these models, they were initially created to explain disparities in health outcomes between whites and Blacks; however, these frameworks have since been expanded to include other historically marginalized communi-ties of color (e.g., Asian American, Latinx; Chou, Asnaani, & Hofmann, 2012).

Based on AL theory, the assessment of indicators of AL varies. For example, among a sample of African American youth, perceived discrimination was associated with higher CRP and BP (Goosby, Malone, Richardson, Cheadle, & Williams, 2015), and higher CRP was found among older African American adults (Lewis, Aiello, Leurgans, Kelly, & Barnes, 2010). Van Dyke and colleagues (2020) examined associations between pervasive discrimination, measured across a variety of settings and situations, and AL via 24 biomarkers (e.g., epinephrine, cortisol, IL-6, CRP) assessing seven physiological systems, namely the HPA, sympathetic response, and cardiovascular system functioning, among a sample of African Americans and whites. Findings revealed greater discrimination was associated with higher AL burden in African Americans (Van Dyke et al., 2020). Also, evidence of AL among Latinx youth, adults, and older adults using indicators including HDL, LDL, CRP, and HbA1c is extensively documented (Gallo et al., 2019; Rodriquez et al., 2019; Salazar et al., 2016). Moreover, in a large multiethnic sample including non-Hispanic Black, Hispanic, and Chinese men and women, everyday discrimination was associated with higher inflammation, measured using IL-6, among women only (Kershaw et al., 2016). Additionally, a longitudinal study among African-American adolescents found those who reported more racial/ethnic discrimination and lower emotional support had higher AL burden (BP, cortisol, catecholamines, epinephrine, norepinephrine, creatinine, and CRP; Brody et al., 2014). Lastly, systematic review evidence echoes these findings, indicating that higher incidence of health risk behaviors and AL disproportionately affect PoC compared to whites (Beckie, 2012; Forde, Crookes, Suglia, & Demmer, 2019; Suvarna et al., 2020). Thus, PoC consistently show increased AL burden compared to whites, which likely results from lifelong and chronic social marginalization and stigma.

Allostatic Load in SGMs

Though this literature is not as established as the PoC literature, theoretical frameworks used to explain AL burden for SGMs is emerging. Meyer's framework (2003) is among the most widely cited minority stress model for SGMs; however, this framework places substantial emphasis on psychological health (Meyer, 2003). Yet, other models explicitly focus on physical health outcomes (Lick, Durso, & Johnson, 2013). Regardless, systematic review evidence links minority stress experienced by SGMs to physical health outcomes, including overall health, immune functioning, cardiovascular health, and HIV risk (Flentje, Heck, Brennan, & Meyer, 2019).

The evidence to date shows greater AL burden in SGMs. For example, in an unpublished dissertation, Outland (2019) examined discrimination and AL as mechanisms to greater rates of chronic health conditions in SGMs over a period of 20 years and found that among gay and bisexual men and women, experiencing greater SGM-related discrimination coupled with greater AL, measured using cortisol, BP, CRP, IL-6, A1c, total cholesterol, and HDL, was associated with more chronic health problems (e.g., cardiovascular diseases [CVDs], cancer). Additionally, Caceres and colleagues (2018) used data from the National Health and Nutrition Examination Survey (NHANES) from 2001 to 2012 and found that lesbian and bisexual women demonstrated an increased risk for CVD through greater BMI and glycosylated hemoglobin compared to heterosexuals. Moreover, DuBois, Powers, Everett, and Juster (2017) examined the relationship between diurnal cortisol functioning and stigma related to the transitioning process among transgender men and found resting cortisol levels were positively associated with transition-based stigma. Also, using data from the NHANES from 2001 to 2010, Mays, Juster, Williamson, Seeman, and Cochran (2018) examined differences among SGM and heterosexuals in AL profiles using nine biomarkers including HDL and CRP. Findings revealed that total AL scores were higher for bisexual men compared to heterosexual men, with gay men demonstrating the lowest levels comparatively (Mays et al., 2018). Thus, an emerging literature base supports the relationship between stress processes salient to SGMs and increased AL burden, which suggests there is a need to focus on racial/ethnic LGBTQ.

Allostatic Load and Intersectional Discrimination

Given the consistent reports of adverse physiological functioning among PoC and SGMs outlined earlier, it is reasonable to suspect that experiences of intersectional discrimination among SGM PoC contribute to adverse physiological health. As discussed in Chap. 2, intentional intersectional frameworks to guide research with SMG PoC are the exception rather than the rule.

While race/ethnicity and sexual orientation–based discrimination are each independently associated with reduced psychological and physiological health, it is apparent that the unique experience of intersectional discrimination matters most for SGM PoC. For example, Fattoracci, Revels-Macalinao, and Huynh (2020) found that the interaction between racism and heterosexism better measured health outcomes including self-reported physical health among a majority Latinx and Asian LGB sample. Further, Caceres, Veldhuis, and Hughes (2019) examined racial/ethnic differences in cardiometabolic risk among SGM women. In their intersectional analyses, Black lesbian and bisexual women were more likely to be obese than White lesbian women. Unexpectedly, however, discrimination (not defined as intersectional) was not significantly associated with adverse health. As a promising study, Rich and colleagues (2020) have released a study protocol for a mixed-method longitudinal study on biopsychosocial mechanisms between SGM stress, CVD, and HIV comorbidity among Black and Latina transgender women, signaling progress in AL research focused exclusively on SGM PoC. Therefore, the literature on AL burden in SGM PoC is growing, but with much yet to be explored.

CONCLUSION

AL provides a useful framework to describe the health consequences of social experiences by capturing the cumulative wear and tear on the body that ultimately produces high disease morbidity, which may result in early mortality for racial/ethnic SGMs. Moreover, AL conceptualizes chronic psychosocial stress and its consequential physiological harm as a catalyst of accelerated physiological aging. Though the existing literature on the AL burden of chronic stress health for PoC is well established, little is known about AL in SGMs, with even less research available to date on AL burden for SGM PoC. Despite this gap, the available literature provides compelling evidence to support the notion that the social marginalization of LGBTQ PoC creates a disproportionate physiological burden. That is, the cumulative nature of intersectional discrimination produces greater AL burden, which subsequently increases risk for negative health outcomes in these communities.

REFERENCES

Beckie, T. M. (2012). A systematic review of allostatic load, health, and health disparities. *Biological Research for Nursing, 14*(4), 311–346. https://doi.org/10.1177/1099800412455688

Brody, G. H., Lei, M. K., Chae, D. H., Yu, T., Kogan, S. M., & Beach, S. R. (2014). Perceived discrimination among African American adolescents and allostatic load: A longitudinal analysis with buffering effects. *Child Development, 85*(3), 989–1002. https://doi.org/10.1111/cdev.12213

Caceres, B. A., Brody, A. A., Halkitis, P. N., Dorsen, C., Yu, G., & Chyun, D. A. (2018). Cardiovascular disease risk in sexual minority women (18–59 years old): Findings from the National Health and Nutrition Examination Survey (2001–2012). *Women's Health Issues, 28*(4), 333–341. https://doi.org/10.1016/j.whi.2018.03.004

Caceres, B. A., Veldhuis, C. B., & Hughes, T. L. (2019). Racial/ethnic differences in cardiometabolic risk in a community sample of sexual minority women. *Health Equity, 3*(1), 350–359. https://doi.org/10.1089/heq.2019.0024

Chou, T., Asnaani, A., & Hofmann, S. G. (2012). Perception of racial discrimination and psychopathology across three US ethnic minority groups. *Cultural Diversity and Ethnic Minority Psychology, 18*(1), 74–81. https://doi.org/10.1037/a0025432

Clark, R., Anderson, N. B., Clark, V., & Williams, D. (1999). Racism as a stressor for African Americans: A biopsychosocial model. *The American Psychologist, 54*(10), 805–816. https://doi.org/10.1037//0003-066x.54.10.805

DuBois, L. Z., Powers, S., Everett, B. G., & Juster, R. P. (2017). Stigma and diurnal cortisol among transitioning transgender men. *Psychoneuroendocrinology, 82*, 59–66. https://doi.org/10.1016/j.psyneuen.2017.05.008

Fattoracci, E. S., Revels-Macalinao, M., & Huynh, Q. L. (2020). Greater than the sum of racism and heterosexism: Intersectional microaggressions toward racial/ethnic and sexual minority group members. *Cultural Diversity and Ethnic Minority Psychology.* https://doi.org/10.1037/cdp0000329

Flentje, A., Heck, N. C., Brennan, J. M., & Meyer, I. H. (2019). The relationship between minority stress and biological outcomes: A systematic review. *Journal of Behavioral Medicine.* https://doi.org/10.1007/s10865-019-00120-6

Forde, A. T., Crookes, D. M., Suglia, S. F., & Demmer, R. T. (2019). The weathering hypothesis as an explanation for racial disparities in health: A systematic review. *Annals of Epidemiology, 33*, 1–18. https://doi.org/10.1016/j.annepidem.2019.02.011

Gallo, L. C., Roesch, S. C., Bravin, J. I., Savin, K. L., Perreira, K., Carnethon, M. R., ... Isasi, C. R. (2019). Socioeconomic adversity, social resources, and allostatic load among Hispanic/Latino youth: The study of Latino youth. *Psychosomatic Medicine, 81*(3), 305–312. https://doi.org/10.1097/PSY.0000000000000668

García, J. J., Serpas, D. G., & Torres, Y. (2020). Taking it to hear: Preliminary investigation on the cardiovascular effects of racial/ethnic microaggressions in Latinx. *Social Behavior Research and. Practice, 5*(1), 1–7. https://doi.org/10.17140/SBRPOJ-5-120

Geronimus, A. (1992). The weathering hypothesis and the health of African-American women and infants: Evidence and speculations. *Ethnicity & Disease*, 2(3), 207–221.

Goosby, B. J., Malone, S., Richardson, E. A., Cheadle, J. E., & Williams, D. T. (2015). Perceived discrimination and markers of cardiovascular risk among low-income African American youth. *American Journal of Human Biology*, 27(4), 546–552. https://doi.org/10.1002/ajhb.22683

Huynh, V. W., Huynh, Q. L., & Stein, M. P. (2017). Not just sticks and stones: Indirect ethnic discrimination leads to greater physiological reactivity. *Cultural Diversity and Ethnic Minority Psychology*, 23(3), 425–434. https://doi.org/10.1037/cdp0000138

Jacobson, R., Cohen, H., & Diamond, G. M. (2016). Gender atypicality and anxiety response to social interaction stress in homosexual and heterosexual men. *Archives of Sexual Behavior*, 45(3), 713–723. https://doi.org/10.1007/s10508-015-0528-y

James, S. A., Hartnett, S. A., & Kalsbeek, W. D. (1983). John Henryism and blood pressure differences among Black men. *Journal of Behavioral Medicine*, 6(3), 259–278. https://doi.org/10.1007/BF01315113

Juster, R. P., Doyle, D. M., Hatzenbuehler, M. L., Everett, B. G., DuBois, L. Z., & McGrath, J. J. (2019). Sexual orientation, disclosure, and cardiovascular stress reactivity. *Stress*, 22(3), 321–331. https://doi.org/10.1080/1025389 0.2019.1579793

Juster, R. P., Hatzenbuehler, M. L., Mendrek, A., Pfaus, J. G., Smith, N. G., Johnson, P. J., ... Pruessner, J. C. (2015). Sexual orientation modulates endocrine stress reactivity. *Biological Psychiatry*, 77(7), 668–676. https://doi.org/10.1016/j.biopsych.2014.08.013

Juster, R. P., McEwen, B. S., & Lupien, S. J. (2010). Allostatic load biomarkers of chronic stress and impact on health and cognition. *Neuroscience & Biobehavioral Reviews*, 35(1), 2–16. https://doi.org/10.1016/j.neubiorev.2009.10.002

Kershaw, K. N., Lewis, T. T., Roux, A. V. D., Jenny, N. S., Liu, K., Peñedo, F. J., & Carnethon, M. R. (2016). Self-reported experiences of discrimination and inflammation among men and women: The Multi-Ethnic Study of Atherosclerosis. *Health Psychology*, 35(4), 343–350. https://doi.org/10.1037/hea0000331

Lewis, T. T., Aiello, A. E., Leurgans, S., Kelly, J., & Barnes, L. L. (2010). Self-reported experiences of everyday discrimination are associated with elevated C-reactive protein levels in older African-American adults. *Brain, Behavior, and Immunity*, 24(3), 438–443. https://doi.org/10.1016/j.bbi.2009.11.011

Lick, D. J., Durso, L. E., & Johnson, K. L. (2013). Minority stress and physical health among sexual minorities. *Perspectives on Psychological Science*, 8(5), 521–548. https://doi.org/10.1177/1745691613497965

Lucas, T., Wegner, R., Pierce, J., Lumley, M. A., Laurent, H. K., & Granger, D. A. (2017). Perceived discrimination, racial identity, and multisystem stress response to social evaluative threat among African American men and women. *Psychosomatic Medicine, 79*(3), 293. https://doi.org/10.1097/PSY.0000000000000406

Mays, V. M., Juster, R. P., Williamson, T. J., Seeman, T. E., & Cochran, S. D. (2018). Chronic physiological effects of stress among lesbian, gay, and bisexual adults: Results from the National Health and Nutrition Examination Survey. *Psychosomatic Medicine, 80*(6), 551–563. https://doi.org/10.1097/PSY.0000000000000600

McEwen, B. S. (1998). Stress, adaptation, and disease: Allostasis and allostatic load. *Annals of the New York Academy of Sciences, 840*(1), 33–44. https://doi.org/10.1111/j.1749-6632.1998.tb09546.x

McEwen, B. S. (2000). The neurobiology of stress: From serendipity to clinical relevance. *Brain Research, 886*(1–2), 172–189. https://doi.org/10.1016/S0006-8993(00)02950-4

McEwen, B. S., & Gianaros, P. J. (2010). Central role of the brain in stress and adaptation: Links to socioeconomic status, health, and disease. *Annals of the New York Academy of Sciences, 1186*, 190–222. https://doi.org/10.1111/j.1749-6632.2009.05331.x

McEwen, B. S., & Stellar, E. (1993). Stress and the individual: Mechanisms leading to disease. *Archives of Internal Medicine, 153*(18), 2093–2101. https://doi.org/10.1001/archinte.1993.00410180039004

Meyer, I. H. (2003). Prejudice, social stress, and mental health in lesbian, gay, and bisexual populations: Conceptual issues and research evidence. *Psychological Bulletin, 129*(5), 674–697. https://doi.org/10.1037/0033-2909.129.5.674

Myers, H. F., Lewis, T. T., & Parker-Dominguez, T. (2003). Stress, coping, and minority health: Biopsychosocial perspective on ethnic health disparities. In G. Bernal, J. E. Trimble, A. K. Burlew, & F. T. L. Leong (Eds.), *Handbook of racial & ethnic minority psychology* (pp. 377–400). SAGE Publications Inc.. https://doi.org/10.4135/9781412976008.n19

Outland, P. (2019). *Biomarkers of allostatic load mediate stress and disease: A prospective structural equation model*. Unpublished doctoral dissertation, Colorado State University.

Parra, L. A., & Hastings, P. D. (2018). Integrating the neurobiology of minority stress with an intersectionality framework for LGBTQ-Latinx populations. *New Directions for Child and Adolescent Development, 161*, 91–108. https://doi.org/10.1002/cad.20244

Rhodes, S. D., Mann-Jackson, L., Alonzo, J., Bell, J. C., Tanner, A. E., Martínez, A. D.,...Brooks, A. R. (2020). The health and well-being of Latinx sexual and gender minorities in the USA: A call to action. In A. D. Martínez & S. D. Rhodes (Eds.), *New and emerging issues in Latinx health* (pp. 217–236). Switzerland: Springer International Publishing. https://doi.org/10.1007/978-3-030-24043-1_10

Rich, A. J., Williams, J., Malik, M., Wirtz, A., Reisner, S., DuBois, ..., & Poteat, T. (2020). Biopsychosocial mechanisms linking gender minority stress to HIV comorbidities among Black and Latina transgender women (LITE plus): Protocol for a mixed methods longitudinal study. *JMIR Research Protocols,* *9*(4), e17076. https://doi.org/10.2196/17076.

Rodriquez, E. J., Sabado-Liwag, M., Pérez-Stable, E. J., Lee, A., Haan, M. N., Gregorich, S. E., ... Nápoles, A. M. (2019). Allostatic load, unhealthy behaviors, and depressive symptoms by birthplace among older adults in the Sacramento area Latino Study on Aging (SALSA). *Journal of Aging and Health.* https://doi.org/10.1177/0898264319857995

Saban, K. L., Mathews, H. L., Bryant, F. B., Tell, D., Joyce, C., DeVon, H. A., & Janusek, L. W. (2018). Perceived discrimination is associated with the inflammatory response to acute laboratory stress in women at risk for cardiovascular disease. *Brain, Behavior, and Immunity, 73,* 625–632. https://doi.org/10.1016/j.bbi.2018.07.010

Salazar, C. R., Strizich, G., Seeman, T. E., Isasi, C. R., Gallo, L. C., Avilés-Santa, L. M., ... Kaplan, R. C. (2016). Nativity differences in allostatic load by age, sex, and Hispanic background from the Hispanic Community Health Study/Study of Latinos. *SSM-Population Health, 2,* 416–424. https://doi.org/10.1016/j.ssmph.2016.05.003

Sawyer, P. J., Major, B., Casad, B. J., Townsend, S. S., & Mendes, W. B. (2012). Discrimination and the stress response: Psychological and physiological consequences of anticipating prejudice in interethnic interactions. *American Journal of Public Health, 102*(5), 1020–1026. https://doi.org/10.2105/AJPH.2011.300620

Sterling, P., & Eyer, J. (1988). Allostasis: A new paradigm to explain arousal pathology. In S. Fisher & J. Reason (Eds.), *Handbook of life stress, cognition and health* (pp. 629–649). John Wiley & Sons.

Suvarna, B., Suvarna, A., Phillips, R., Juster, R. P., McDermott, B., & Sarnyai, Z. (2020). Health risk behaviours and allostatic load: A systematic review. *Neuroscience & Biobehavioral Reviews, 108,* 694–711. https://doi.org/10.1016/j.neubiorev.2019.12.020

Van Dyke, M. E., Baumhofer, N. K. I., Slopen, N., Mujahid, M. S., Clark, C. R., Williams, D. R., & Lewis, T. T. (2020). Pervasive discrimination and allostatic load in African American and White adults. *Psychosomatic Medicine, 82*(3), 316–323. https://doi.org/10.1097/PSY.0000000000000788

PART II

LGBTQ PoC Heart Health

CHAPTER 5

Cardiovascular Disease Risk Factor Burden in LGBTQ PoC

James J. García and Dylan G. Serpas

Abstract Despite emerging evidence of LGBTQ heart health disparities, few studies focus on racial/ethnic LGBTQ. Cardiovascular diseases (Cvds) are the leading causes of morbidity and mortality in the United States. There are separate bodies of literature indicating there are modifiable cardiovascular risk factor disparities among racial/ethnic and sexual minority/gender-diverse people. However, what is missing is an intersectional focus on risk factor differences, which may shed light on differential risk for Cvds among racial/ethnic LGBTQ. Guided by the minority stress theory, this chapter focuses on how minority stress (in the form of intersectional discrimination) is a possible pathway for CVD risk for LGBTQ people of color (PoC). Thus, this chapter focuses on the small, yet emerging,

J. J. García (✉)
Department of Psychology, School of Health and Community Well-Being, University of La Verne, La Verne, CA, USA
e-mail: JGarcia4@laverne.edu

D. G. Serpas
Department of Psychology, California State University, Fullerton, Fullerton, CA, USA

J. J. García (ed.), *Heart, Brain and Mental Health Disparities for LGBTQ People of Color*, https://doi.org/10.1007/978-3-030-70060-7_5

55

literature on CVDs for LGBTQ PoC, with a centering of the associations of intersectional discrimination with CVD health for these communities.

Keywords CVDs • Intersectionality • Risk Factors

Although there is emerging evidence of LGBTQ heart health disparities in the research, few studies focus on racial/ethnic LGBTQ. Cardiovascular diseases (CVDs) are the leading causes of morbidity and mortality in the United States (Virani et al., 2020). There are separate bodies of literature that indicate there are modifiable cardiovascular risk factor (CVD RF) disparities among racial/ethnic (Virani et al., 2020) and sexual minority/gender-diverse people (Caceres et al., 2017). However, what is missing is an intersectional focus (i.e., examining risk factors in LGBTQ people of color [PoC]) on CVD RF differences, which may shed light on differential risk for CVDs for racial/ethnic LGBTQ. Guided by the minority stress theory (MST; Meyer, 2003), this chapter will focus on explicating how minority stress (in the form of intersectional discrimination) is a possible pathway for CVD risk for LGBTQ PoC. Moreover, guided by the allostatic load framework, this chapter will detail the CVD RF burden on LGBTQ PoC and help conceptualize how the repeated wear and tear of the body, resulting from chronic experiences of intersectional discrimination, may lead to deleterious CVD health for LGBTQ PoC. Thus, this chapter focuses on the small, yet emerging, empirical literature on CVD RFs for LGBTQ PoC, including studies focused on the associations of intersectional discrimination with CVD RFs.

In the United States, CVDs rank among the current top three leading causes of death (Centers for Disease Control and Prevention, 2019). CVDs develop from the accumulation of CVD RFs over the life span (Hardy, Lawlor, & Kuh, 2015). Across the world, evidence from the multisite INTERHEART Study of 52 countries shows that potentially modifiable CVD-related psychosocial and bio-behavioral factors account for a substantial risk for heart attacks (Yusuf et al., 2004). Moreover, extensive and consistent epidemiological data show disproportionately higher CVD RF burden for PoC compared to whites in the United States (Virani et al., 2020); these findings mirror the greater prevalence, incidence, and mortality for CVDs in racial/ethnic communities compared to white LGBTQ. In a separate line of research, emerging data indicate LGBTQ people experience greater CVD RF burden compared to cisgender and heterosexual counterparts (Caceres et al., 2017; Caceres, Veldhuis, & Hughes, 2019). These findings are in the context of national data indicating the United States will become a majority racial/ethnic country by 2055 (U.S. Census Bureau, 2016), with a sizeable population (4.5%) identifying as LGBTQ (Gallup, 2018). Thus, there is a pressing need to examine CVD burden for racial/ethnic LGBTQ communities.

Despite concerning CVD findings, the majority of leading health research and funding for LGBTQ health focuses on Human Immunodeficiency Virus (HIV) infection and/or Acquired Immune Deficiency Syndrome (AIDS; Coulter, Kenst, Bowen,, & Scout, 2014). Importantly, 68.6% of all NIH-funded studies fail to report race/ethnicity of their sample, which precludes an examination of RF burden for racial/ethnic LGBTQ in the context of CVD health (Coulter et al., 2014, p. 110). Thus, identifying CVD RF burden for LGBTQ PoC has the potential to directly inform medical and psychosocial intervention strategies aimed at reducing cardiovascular health risk and promote health equity for racial/ethnic LGBTQ communities in the United States.

CVD BIO-BEHAVIORAL RISK FACTORS

Central to CVD are health behaviors, or actions, carried out by an individual that negatively impact CVD health (Yusuf et al., 2004). These bio-behavioral factors, that is behavioral factors that impact biology, can be divided into modifiable or non-modifiable. Examples of modifiable risk bio-behavioral factors include smoking and alcohol use, whereas non-modifiable risk factors include age.

Evidence shows deleterious health behaviors increase CVD RF burden for PoC, which result in high prevalence, incidence, and mortality from CVD (Virani et al., 2020). For example, smoking accounts for 36% of risk (PAR), whereas alcohol use has a 13.9% of risk for myocardial infarctions (Yusuf et al., 2004). Separately, recent systematic review evidence demonstrates a disproportionate CVD bio-behavioral burden for LGBTQ communities compared to cisgender/heterosexual counterparts (Caceres et al., 2017; Caceres, Veldhuis, & Hughes, 2019). However, the majority of studies focus on either PoC or LGBTQ populations, which precludes any examination of bio-behavioral factors that influence CVD health of those who identify as LGBTQ PoC. Indeed, several scholars have called for an intersectionality focus in the study of racial/ethnic LGBTQ health (Bowleg, 2012; Cyrus, 2017), including in the CVD health literature

(Ruiz & Brondolo, 2016). Therefore, there is a need for data on modifiable CVD RFs for LGBTQ PoC, as these are important targets for psychosocial interventions. The following section will present broad LGB CVD-related modifiable bio-behavioral factors, explore findings with transgender and gender-non-conforming communities, and highlight specific racial/ethnic LGBTQ data disaggregated by race/ethnicity when possible.

TRADITIONAL CVD RF BURDEN IN SEXUAL MINORITIES

Few studies focus on assessing traditional CVD RFs among sexual minorities; however, most are assessed via self-report and few use objective assessments for RFs. Whenever possible, the following section will denote when self-report or objective CVD RF assessments were used. With regard to self-report body mass index (BMI), sexual minority men (e.g., gay and bisexual men) were less likely to self-report being overweight or obese; however, sexual minority women (i.e., lesbian and bisexual women) were more likely to report being overweight or obese when compared to their heterosexual counterparts (Caceres et al., 2017); this is consistent with secondary analyses National Health and Nutrition Examination Survey (NHANES) 2001–2012 (Caceres et al., 2018) and the 2014–2016 Behavioral Risk Factor Surveillance System (BRFSS; Caceres, Jackman, Edmondson, & Bockting, 2019). Their review also found most studies used self-reported CVD diagnoses, with sexual minority women indicating greater CVD diagnoses in three studies and gay men under 40 reporting increased diagnosis of CVD in one study (Caceres et al., 2017); the former findings are partly consistent with findings from the 2014–2016 BRFSS (Caceres et al., 2019). In terms of race/ethnicity, Latinx and Black lesbian and bisexual women demonstrated the highest overweight and obesity rates compared to their heterosexual PoC and white LGBTQ counterparts (Caceres et al., 2017). Taken together, an elevated CVD RF burden for lesbian and bisexual LGBTQ in BMI and CVD diagnoses is evident, with Latinx lesbian and bisexual women having the highest rates of greater BMI.

CVD RF Burden in LGB PoC

The systematic review by Caceres et al. (2017) is the most up-to-date and closest estimate of CVD health with LGB persons, with all comparisons made to heterosexual male and female counterparts of the same race/

ethnicity. Regarding bio-behavioral factors, Caceres and colleagues found that gay and bisexual men had significantly higher self-report tobacco use and this trend was also observed in lesbian and bisexual women; the former is in line the 2014–2016 BRFSS, where gay men had elevated smoking rates (Caceres, Veldhuis, & Hughes, 2019). In terms of racial/ethnic differences, their systematic review found four studies showing tobacco use was significantly higher only among lesbian and bisexual Latina women. In a recent study, minority stress was associated with greater likelihood of current smoking across middle and older age cohorts of Black and Latino LGB persons in the Generations Study (Gordon et al., 2020). Next, self-reported alcohol consumption was found as the highest among lesbian and bisexuals; however, a further parsing of the data showed Latina lesbian and bisexual women reporting significantly greater alcohol use, consistent with a secondary analyses of the NHANES from 2001–2012 (Caceres et al., 2018), the fourth wave of the National Longitudinal Study of Adolescent to Adult Health (i.e., ADD Health; Goldberg, Conron, & Halpern, 2019), and the 2014–2016 BRFSS (Caceres, Jackman, et al., 2019). From these data, a consistent finding is an elevated risk factor burden in LGB samples, yet there is limited representation of racial/ethnic LGB persons, as only four studies to date identified within the context of CVD RF burden. Thus, there appears to be a disproportionately greater burden of alcohol and tobacco use for Latinx lesbian and bisexual women in the context of CVDs.

Objective CVD RF Burden in LGB PoC

The systematic review by Caceres et al. (2017) identified studies using objective CVD biomarkers, including blood pressure, heart rate, and C-reactive protein. Overall, sexual minority men and women had an increased risk of objective CVD risk factors. In particular, four studies used objective blood pressure readings and found that gay men were two times more likely to have objective hypertension. These findings are corroborated with findings for sexual minority men in the NHANES 2001–2012 (Caceres et al., 2018). Among lesbian and bisexual women, only two studies found greater risk for objectively assessed hypertension. With diabetes, only one study found objectively higher rates of diabetes in gay and bisexual men, whereas two studies indicate bisexual women are more likely to self-report a history of diabetes; the latter is consistent with a secondary analysis of the NHANES 2001–2012 (Caceres et al., 2018).

Lastly, one study found objectively higher cholesterol in gay and bisexual men, and one study demonstrated objectively lower cholesterol among lesbian and bisexual women.

To this end, in a unique analysis of lesbian, gay, and bisexual PoC from the 2001–2016 NHANES of over 22,000 participants, Caceres et al. (2020) found Black bisexual women showed higher objectively assessed BMI, greater systolic blood pressure (SBP), and higher HbA1c compared to white heterosexual women; Black sexual minority men had elevated objectively assessed HbA1c compared to heterosexual men; Latinos who identified their sexual orientation as "not sure" had objectively assessed greater SBP, higher HbA1c, and total cholesterol. As demonstrated, there is disproportionate CVD RF burden in sexual minority communities. Yet, few studies rely on objective assessments of CVD RFs, with even fewer focusing specifically on racial/ethnic LGB people. Thus, research focused on objective CVD RF burden in racial/ethnic LGB is sorely needed.

CVD RF Burden in Gender-Diverse People

Despite an emerging and recent interest in sexual minority CVD health, there are very few studies focused on CVD RF burden for gender-diverse people; that is, Transgender and Gender-Non-conforming (TGNC) persons. Often, TGNC have little to no representation in the scientific literature; this further marginalizes and perpetuates systemic oppression for these communities. To this end, this section highlights data on TGNC persons and what is known about CVD health and health disparities for these communities, highlighting studies on Black and Latinx transgender communities.

In a narrative review, Streed et al. (2017) found differential CVD health risk for transgender men and women receiving gender-affirming hormone therapy, such that transgender women (but not trans men) demonstrated greater CVD RF burden. However, a recent analysis of transwomen and men from federally qualified health centers across the U.S. found that gender-affirming hormone therapy was not associated with hypertension risk, but recent progestin prescription was associated with a diagnosis of thromboembolism (i.e., blood clot that becomes dislodged and clogs a blood vessel). In light of these findings, an analysis of the 2014–2017 BRFSS of 1373 transgender men, 570 transgender women, and 570 GNC persons by Caceres, Veldhuis, and Hughes (2019) found (compared to cisgender men and women) transgender men and women were more likely to be overweight; transgender women had greater rates of diabetes, angina/coronary heart disease, strokes, and myocardial infarction (MI) and reporting any CVD; transgender men had greater odds of reporting a stroke; GNC persons had greater rates of MI; and significantly greater tobacco use emerged for transgender men and women. Worthy to note, findings from the Caceres et al. study have been replicated by Alzahrani et al. (2019) given they used the same dataset, namely increased MI risk for transgender women; however, other findings were not consistent despite both research groups using the same dataset. This finding may be partly due to Alzahrani et al. not including those who identified as GNC. Worthy to note, these studies are the comparisons of gender minorities of both cisgender men and women groups; however, these data are not stratified by race/ethnicity, despite the fact that racial/ethnic TGNC people composed about 30% of the total TGNC sample. Thus, results shed some light on the TGNC CVD RF profile, but they also indicate that further research is needed to clarify CVD RF burden for gender-diverse PoC.

CVD RF Burden in Racial/Ethnic TGNC

As illustrated, there are relatively few studies that exclusively focus on CVD RF burden in TGNC persons, with even fewer available that examine racial/ethnic LGBTQ. Nonetheless, there are glimmers of racial/ethnic CVD RF burden in existing literature. For example, an examination of CVD RF burden within the context of HIV by Gogia et al. (2018) used a hospital-based registry of over 5000 people in the Boston area (with 55% of the sample identifying as Black and Latinx) and found that transgender women with HIV (compared to cisgender men with HIV) had higher diabetes prevalence. However, this study is within the context of HIV and data are not parsed out by race/ethnicity, despite the large racial/ethnic composition of the sample. In another study including racial/ethnic TGNC persons, Cabrera-Serrano, Felici-Giovanini, Diaz-Toro, and Cases-Rosario (2014) examined the Puerto Rico BRFFS and found greater self-reported cholesterol, hypertension, CVD diagnosis, diabetes, and BMI for the collapsed LGBTQ group comprised of 4132 Latinx heterosexual transgender and 564 bisexual transgender persons. However, their analyses focused on differences between smokers and nonsmokers and results collapsed TGNC persons with sexual minority people. To add further complexity, an international study of transgender women in Lima, Peru, found that increased stimulant use (i.e., cocaine use) accounted for 15% of CVD mortality (Bórquez et al., 2020). An ongoing study with a published protocol by Rich et al. (2020) will examine CVD RFs in the context of HIV for 200 Black and transgender women. Their mixed-methods study protocol will focus on examining longitudinal CVD RFs for Black and Latinx transwomen living with HIV to understand comorbidity. Despite that data are not yet available, this study highlights an instance of where researchers examine CVD RFs in the context of HIV; though helpful, this perpetuates further stigmatization by conflating racial/ethnic LGBTQ persons with HIV and precludes an ability to examine the CVD RF burden on Black and Latinx transpersons living without HIV. Thus, studies that have an explicit focus on CVD RF burden and that center racial/ethnic LGBTQ are the exception rather than the rule.

INTERSECTIONAL DISCRIMINATION AND CVD RISK FOR LGBTQ PoC

One psychosocial stressor salient to Latinx and Black LGBTQ, with growing evidence as a unique and distinctive pathway in the development of CVD health disparities, is intersectional discrimination (Balsam, Molina, Beadnell, Simoni, & Walters, 2011; Scheim & Bauer, 2019). This contextual factor reflects the unique lived experiences of persons who hold several unique racial/ethnic and sexual and gender minority identities, including interlocking dynamics of power, privilege, oppression, and marginalization experienced in the form of minority stress at the societal/systemic and individual levels (Hendricks & Testa, 2012; Meyer & Frost, 2013). Despite substantial evidence linking experiences of discrimination for marginalized identities to negative physical health outcomes (Pascoe & Smart Richman, 2009), studies examining intersectional discrimination (both blatant or subtle) and CVD RF burden in LGBTQ PoC are virtually nonexistent. This is surprising, given the substantive qualitative research to date focused on intersectional microaggression for LGBTQ PoC (Nadal et al., 2017).

Similar to racism as a unique psychosocial stressor for communities of color (Brondolo, Brady, Libby, & Pencille, 2011) acting via an acute cardiovascular reactivity (CVR) pathway that increases CVD risk (Treiber et al., 2003), intersectional discrimination—as psychosocial experience that increases allostatic load—may function through this similar CVR pathway for LGBTQ PoC. To date, studies with LGB people indicate minority stress functions via a CVR pathway (Juster et al., 2019). As suggested by Shangani, Gamarel, Ogunbajo, Cai, and Operario (2020), intersectional discrimination is a unique and chronic form of minority stress experienced to a greater degree among LGBTQ PoC (namely Black and Latinx gay and bisexual men and women) compared to White LGB. Moreover, evidence suggests intersectional discrimination acts as a chronic, traumatic and oppressive stressor for marginalized communities (Holmes, Facemire, & DaFonseca, 2016). In the only study to date examining intersectional discrimination and CVD health of LGBTQ PoC, Caceres, Jackman, et al. (2019) examined 601 lesbian and bisexual women of color and tested the association between discrimination and CVD RFs. They found that Black lesbian and Black bisexual persons were more likely to be obese and Black lesbians were more likely to report a history of hypertension and diabetes. However, their findings suggest discrimination was not associated with CVD health; the discrimination assessment used did not specify which identities were targeted, whether questions assessed blatant or subtle discrimination, relied on self-report CVD RFs, and did not include gender minorities of color. Thus, intersectional discrimination may operate through an acute CVR pathway, thereby increasing CVD risk for LGBTQ PoC; however, this literature is in its infancy and is slowly emerging.

Summary

As evidenced in this chapter, there are very few studies that examine differences in CVD RF burden or CVD mortality for LGBTQ PoC. Moreover, few discuss the role of intersectional discrimination as a psychosocial stress pathway that increases risk for CVD burden for racial/ethnic LGBTQ; this is in sharp contrast to the sizeable literature of racism as a psychosocial risk factor for CVD health in heterosexual communities of color. Of note, of the studies that examine racial/ethnic LGBTQ, frequent comparisons are made to White LGBTQ as comparisons. Using this methodology does a disservice to racial/ethnic LGBTQ, as it compares communities who have faced historical disadvantage to groups with power and privilege; though helpful for health disparities research, this approach does not center or explore CVD health within racial/ethnic LGBTQ persons before comparisons to White LGBTQ are made. Additionally, the limited literature with transgender people conflates CVD with HIV, with some in the context of gender-affirming hormone therapy; this suggests there is a need to examine general CVD health for racial/ethnic transgender men and women pre-hormone therapy and living without HIV to understand baseline CVD health burden. Moving forward, there is a significant need to center racial/ethnic LGBTQ in studies of CVD health disparities to promote health equity for these communities.

REFERENCES

Alzahrani, T., Nguyen, T., Ryan, A., Dwairy, A., McCaffrey, J., Yunus, R., ..., & Reiner, J. (2019). Cardiovascular disease risk factors and myocardial infarction in the transgender population. *Circulation: Cardiovascular Quality and Outcomes*, *12*(4), e005597. https://doi.org/10.1161/CIRCOUT COMES.119.005597.

Balsam, K. F., Molina, Y., Beadnell, B., Simoni, J., & Walters, K. (2011). Measuring multiple minority stress: The LGBT People of Color Microaggressions Scale. *Cultural Diversity and Ethnic Minority Psychology*, *17*(2), 163–174. https://doi.org/10.1037/a0023244

Bórquez, A., Rich, K., Farrell, M., Degenhardt, L., McKetin, R., Tran, L. T., ... Kelly, S. (2020). Integrating HIV pre-exposure prophylaxis and harm reduction among men who have sex with men and transgender women to address intersecting harms associated with stimulant use: A modelling study. *Journal of the International AIDS Society*, *23*(S1), e25495. https://doi.org/10.1002/jia2.25495

Bowleg, L. (2012). The problem with the phrase women and minorities: Intersectionality—An important theoretical framework for public health. *American Journal of Public Health*, *102*(7), 1267–1273. https://doi.org/10.2105/AJPH.2012.300750

Brondolo, E., Brady, N., Libby, D. J., & Pencille, M. (2011). Racism as a psychosocial stressor. In R. J. Contrada & A. Baum (Eds.), *Handbook of stress science: Biology, psychology, and health* (pp. 167–184). New York, NY: Springer Publishing Company.

Cabrera-Serrano, A., Felici-Giovanini, M. E., Diaz-Toro, E. C., & Cases-Rosario, A. L. (2014). Disproportionate tobacco use in the Puerto Rico lesbian, gay, bisexual, and transgender community of 18 years and over—A descriptive profile. *LGBT Health*, *1*(2), 107–112. https://doi.org/10.1089/lgbt.2013.0011

Caceres, B. A., Ancheta, A. J., Dorsen, C., Newlin-Lew, K., Edmondson, D., & Hughes, T. L. (2020). A population-based study of the intersection of sexual identity and race/ethnicity on physiological risk factors for CVD among US adults (ages 18–59). *Ethnicity & Health*, *11*, 1–22. https://doi.org/10.108 0/13557858.2020.1740174.

Caceres, B. A., Brody, A., Luscombe, R. E., Primiano, J. E., Marusca, P., Sitts, E. M., et al. (2017). A systematic review of cardiovascular disease in sexual minorities. *American Journal of Public Health, 107*(4), e13–e21. https://doi.org/10.2105/AJPH.2016.303630

Caceres, B. A., Brody, A. A., Halkitis, P. N., Dorsen, C., Yu, G., & Chyun, D. A. (2018). Cardiovascular disease risk in sexual minority women (18–59 years old): Findings from the National Health and Nutrition Examination Survey (2001–2012). *Women's Health Issues, 28*(4), 333–341. https://doi.org/10.1016/j.whi.2018.03.004

Caceres, B. A., Jackman, K. B., Edmondson, D., & Bockting, W. O. (2019). Assessing gender identity differences in cardiovascular disease in US adults: An analysis of data from the 2014–2017 BRFSS. *Journal of Behavioral Medicine, 43*, 1–10. https://doi.org/10.1007/s10865-019-00102-8

Caceres, B. A., Veldhuis, C. B., & Hughes, T. L. (2019). Racial/ethnic differences in cardiometabolic risk in a community sample of sexual minority women. *Health Equity, 3*(1), 350–359. https://doi.org/10.1089/heq.2019.0024

Centers for Disease Control and Prevention. (2019). Leading causes of death. Retrieved from https://www.cdc.gov/nchs/fastats/leading-causes-of-death.htm.

Coulter, R. W. S., Kenst, K. S., Bowen, D. J., & Scout. (2014). Research funded by the National Institutes of Health on the health of lesbian, gay, bisexual, and transgender populations. *American Journal of Public Health, 104*(2), 105–112. https://doi.org/10.2105/AJPH.2013.301501

Cyrus, K. (2017). Multiple minorities as multiply marginalized: Applying the minority stress theory to LGBTQ people of color. *Journal of Gay & Lesbian Mental Health, 21*(3), 194–202. https://doi.org/10.1080/1935970 5.2017.1320739

Gallup. (2018). U.S. estimates of LGBT population rises to 4.5%. https://news.gallup.com/poll/234863/estimate-lgbt-population-rises.aspx.

Gogia, S., Coromilas, A., Regan, S., Stone, L., Fourman, L. T., Triant, V. A., ... Zanni, M. V. (2018). Cardiovascular risk profile of transgender women with HIV: A US healthcare database study. *Journal of Acquired Immune Deficiency Syndromes, 79*(1), e39–e41. https://doi.org/10.1097/QAI.00000 00000001767

Goldberg, S. K., Conron, K. J., & Halpern, C. T. (2019). Metabolic syndrome and economic strain among sexual minority young adults. *LGBT Health, 6*(1), 1–8. https://doi.org/10.1089/lgbt.2018.0053

Gordon, A. R., Fish, J. N., Kiekens, W. J., Lightfoot, M., Frost, D. M., & Russell, S. T. (2020). Cigarette smoking and minority stress across age cohorts in a national sample of sexual minorities: Results from the Generations Study. *Annals of Behavioral Medicine*, kaaa079. https://doi.org/10.1093/abm/kaaa079.

Hardy, R., Lawlor, D. A., & Kuh, D. (2015). A life course approach to cardiovascular aging. *Future Cardiology, 11*(1), 101–113. https://doi.org/10.2217/FCA.14.67

Hendricks, M. L., & Testa, R. J. (2012). A conceptual framework for clinical work with transgender and gender nonconforming clients: An adaptation of the minority stress model. *Professional Psychology: Research and Practice, 43*(5), 460–467. https://doi.org/10.1037/a0029597

Holmes, S. C., Facemire, V. C., & DaFonseca, A. M. (2016). Expanding criterion a for posttraumatic stress disorder: Considering the deleterious impact of oppression. *Traumatology, 22*(4), 314. https://doi.org/10.1037/trm0000104

Juster, R. P., Doyle, D. M., Hatzenbuehler, M. L., Everett, B. G., DuBois, L. Z., & McGrath, J. J. (2019). Sexual orientation, disclosure, and cardiovascular stress reactivity. *Stress, 22*(3), 321–331. https://doi.org/10.1080/1025389 0.2019.1579793

Meyer, I. H. (2003). Prejudice, social stress, and mental health in lesbian, gay, and bisexual populations: conceptual issues and research evidence. *Psychological Bulletin, 129*(5), 674. https://doi.org/10.1037/0033-2909.129.5.674

Meyer, I. H., & Frost, D. M. (2013). Minority stress and the health of sexual minorities. In C. J. Patterson & A. R. D'Augelli (Eds.), *Handbook of psychology and sexual orientation* (pp. 252–266). Oxford University Press.

Nadal, K. L., Erazo, T., Schulman, J., Han, H., Deutsch, T., Ruth, R., & Santacruz, E. (2017). Caught at the intersections: Microaggressions toward lesbian, gay, bisexual, transgender, and queer people of color. In R. Ruth & E. Santacruz (Eds.), *LGBTQ psychology and mental health: Emerging research and advances* (pp. 133–152). ABC-CLIO, LLC.

Pascoe, E. A., & Smart Richman, L. (2009). Perceived discrimination and health: A meta-analytic review. *Psychological Bulletin, 135*(4), 531–554. https://doi.org/10.1037/a0016059

Rich, A. J., Williams, J., Malik, M., Wirtz, A., Reisner, S., DuBois, L. Z., … Cannon, C. (2020). Biopsychosocial mechanisms linking gender minority stress to HIV comorbidities among Black and Latina Transgender Women (LITE Plus): Protocol for a mixed methods longitudinal study. *JMIR Research Protocols, 9*(4), e17076. https://doi.org/10.2196/17076

Ruiz, J. M., & Brondolo, E. (2016). Introduction to the special issue disparities in cardiovascular health: Examining the contributions of social and behavioral factors. *Health Psychology, 35*(4), 309. https://doi.org/10.1037/hea0000364

Scheim, A. I., & Bauer, G. R. (2019). The intersectional discrimination index: Development and validation of measures of self-reported enacted and anticipated discrimination for intercategorical analysis. *Social Science & Medicine, 226*, 225–235. https://doi.org/10.1016/j.socscimed.2018.12.016

Shangani, S., Gamarel, K. E., Ogunbajo, A., Cai, J., & Operario, D. (2020). Intersectional minority stress disparities among sexual minority adults in the USA: The role of race/ethnicity and socioeconomic status. *Culture, Health & Sexuality, 22*(4), 398–412. https://doi.org/10.1080/1369105 8.2019.1604994

Streed Jr, C. G., Harfouch, O., Marvel, F., Blumenthal, R. S., Martin, S. S., & Mukherjee, M. (2017). Cardiovascular disease among transgender adults receiving hormone therapy: a narrative review. *Annals of internal medicine, 167*(4), 256–267. https://doi.org/10.7326/M17-0577

Treiber, F. A., Kamarck, T., Schneiderman, N., Sheffield, D., Kapuku, G., & Taylor, T. (2003). Cardiovascular reactivity and development of preclinical and clinical disease states. *Psychosomatic Medicine, 65*(1), 46–62.

United States Census Bureau. (2016). New census bureau report analyzes U.S. population projections. Retrieved from https://www.census.gov/news-room/press-releases/2015/cb15-tps16.html

Virani, S. S., Alonso, A., Benjamin, E. J., Bittencourt, M. S., Callaway, C. W., Carson, A. P., ... Djousse, L. (2020). Heart disease and stroke statistics—2020 update: A report from the American Heart Association. *Circulation,* E139–E596. https://doi.org/10.1161/CIR.0000000000000757

Yusuf, S., Hawken, S., Ôunpuu, S., Dans, T., Avezum, A., Lanas, F., ... & Lisheng, L. (2004). Effect of potentially modifiable risk factors associated with myocardial infarction in 52 countries (the INTERHEART study): Case-control study. *The Lancet, 364*(9438), 937–952. https://doi.org/10.1016/S0140-6736(04)17018-9

CHAPTER 6

Comorbid Cardiovascular Diseases and HIV in LGBTQ PoC

Maleeha Abbas and James J. García

Abstract Cardiovascular diseases (CVDs) are the leading cause of deaths worldwide. Data suggest people who identify as sexual/gender minorities (SGMs) or LGBTQ have greater CVD risk due to experiences of social marginalization compared to heterosexual counterparts. Parallel to this, evidence suggests People of Color (PoC) have an elevated risk for CVDs compared to White individuals. In addition to high CVD burden, LGBTQ PoC are also disproportionately affected by the human immunodeficiency virus (HIV). This chapter details the comorbidity of heart disease and HIV. Moreover, psychosocial risk factors (RFs) overlapping with heart disease and HIV are highlighted. The chapter ends by exploring the role of intersectional discrimination, HIV, and heart disease.

M. Abbas (✉)
Department of Psychology, University of La Verne, La Verne, CA, USA
e-mail: maleeha.abbas@laverne.edu;

J. J. García
Department of Psychology, School of Health and Community Well-Being, University of La Verne, La Verne, CA, USA
e-mail: JGarcia4@laverne.edu

J. J. García (ed.), *Heart, Brain and Mental Health Disparities for LGBTQ People of Color*,
https://doi.org/10.1007/978-3-030-70060-7_6

69

Keywords CVDs and HIV • Intersectional Discrimination • Social
Marginalization

Cardiovascular diseases (CVDs) are the leading cause of deaths worldwide
(Biglu, Ghavami, & Biglu, 2016; World Health Organization, 2017) and
include disorders of the heart and blood vessels such as arrhythmias, coronary heart disease, heart attack, high blood pressure, congenital heart
defects, vascular dementia, and stroke (National Heart, Lung, and Blood
Institute, 2020). Data suggest people who identify as sexual/gender minorities (SGMs), or LGBTQ, have greater CVD risk due to experiences of
social marginalization compared to heterosexual counterparts (Caceres
et al., 2017). Parallel to this, evidence suggests People of Color (PoC) have
an elevated risk for CVDs compared to White individuals (Virani et al., 2020).

   In addition to high CVD burden, LGBTQ PoC are also disproportionately affected by the human immunodeficiency virus (HIV). This disease
process targets immune system cells, resulting in a progressive deterioration of the body's immune defense system (World Health Organization,
2017), affecting over 34 million people around the globe (Stevens, Lynm,
& Golub, 2012). The World Health Organization (2017) recognizes that
HIV-infected patients are best managed within a chronic disease framework (Mahungu, Rodger, & Johnson, 2009). Often, people who are
infected with HIV are treated with highly active antiretroviral therapy
(HAART), which reduces the risk of death (WHO, 2017). Strong evidence
suggests HIV disproportionately affects LGBT PoC. In particular, the
Centers of Disease Control indicates that gay and bisexual men accounted
for 64% of new HIV diagnoses in the United States, with 70% identifying
as PoC, including Hispanic/Latino, Black/African-American, Asian, and
American Indians (CDC, 2017). Together, high burden of HIV and CVD
is experienced by LGBTQ and PoC, which makes the examination of
comorbid HIV and CVD in SGMs of Color (SGMoC) a priority.

How Are HIV and CVD Related?

With the introduction of HAART, better survival rates have been demonstrated; however, PLWH are developing high risk of comorbid diseases of
aging, namely noncommunicable diseases like CVDs (Chow et al., 2012).
Research shows that people living with HIV (PLWH) have a greater prevalence rate of hypertension and CVDs (Smit, Cassidy, & Cozzi-Lepri,
2017). More specifically, data suggest that HIV infection is linked with

increased risk for acute myocardial infarction, heart failure, and ischemic stroke (Freiberg et al., 2013).

The risk of CVD observed in HIV-infected patients has been attributed to a variety of behavioral and biological factors. Growing literature has examined the associations of HIV infection and CVD risk factors (RFs), even in patients who have undetectable viral load (Kaplan, Hanna, & Kizer, 2016). For example, the National Heart, Lung, and Blood Institute (NHLBI) HIV-CVD collaborative found that among young PLWH, carotid intima–media thickness (a subclinical indicator of atherosclerosis, a form of coronary heart disease) was present in those who were HIV-positive, with systolic blood pressure and lower high-density lipoproteins increasing with age (Hanna et al., 2016). Moreover, a review of the data with PLWH in the post-HAART era indicates HIV infection is associated with higher risk for other CVDs outside CHD, including heart failure, stroke, and arrhythmias; this suggests chronic inflammation may be an underlying mechanism in producing increased CVD burden even when HIV is well controlled (Barnes, Lacson, & Bahrami, 2017). In terms of health behaviors, PLWH demonstrate higher smoking rates than the general population (Saves et al., 2003). Despite no direct correlation between cigarette smoking and HIV acquisition, data show that greater smoking use in bisexual Black youth (Feinstein et al., 2019) is associated with increased risk of CVDs and of contracting HIV among sexual and gender minorities (Morgan et al., 2016). Additionally, being overweight is a RF for developing CVD in PLWH, in addition to HIV medications producing this side effect (Obry-Roguet et al., 2018), and this has been documented in transgender PLWH and in risk for CVDs (Smeaton et al., 2020). Therefore, increase risk of CVDs in PLWH may be due to direct consequences of HIV infection (i.e., inflammation; Barnes et al., 2017), side effects of HAART medications (Nsagha et al., 2015), and the shared bio-behavioral RFs between HIV and CVDs (So-Armah & Freiberg, 2014).

Heightened CVD risk burden in PLWH has led some scholars to recognize HIV infection as a traditional CVD RFs, given that it is similar in magnitude to other traditional RFs such as smoking, hypertension, diabetes, and lipids (Hsue & Waters, 2018). This call to research has mobilized the scientific community to develop innovative research on CVDs in the context of HIV. For example, the ImPlementation REsearCh to DEvelop Interventions for People Living with HIV (the PRECluDe consortium) is using innovative implementation agendas with mental health, HIV, cardiovascular, and pulmonary health to enhance HIV and chronic disease management. In particular, they have updated the HIV treatment cascade model by adding a stage where patients are assessed for any high cholesterol, coronary syndrome, peripheral arterial disease, myocardial infarction, and stroke (Gamble-George et al., 2020). Moreover, the Randomized Trial to Prevent Vascular Events in HIV (REPRIEVE) in over five continents has undertaken the monumental task of preventing CVDs through statins in PLWH who are receiving HAART (Grinspoon, Douglas, Hoffmann, & Ribaudo, 2020). The REPRIEVE study is a promising trial, as it will be reflective of the racial/ethnic, sexual/gender diversity across the globe. Thus, research is moving in the direction of acknowledging and addressing the comorbidity of CVDs for PLWH.

PSYCHOSOCIAL RISK FACTORS IN HIV AND CVD

People living with HIV require great emotional support as it relates to coping with their status and existing in a society as an HIV-positive person (Gerbi, Habtemariam, Robnett, Nganwa, & Tameru, 2012). This is because HIV is a socially stigmatized disease that impacts a person's ability to secure unemployment, housing, and financial stability, and to maintain romantic/sexual relationships (Gerbi et al., 2012). Moreover, evidence indicates depression and psychosocial stress are associated with subclinical atherosclerosis in PLWH (Levy et al., 2020).

As a psychosocial stressor, the unique experiences of anti-LGBTQ rhetoric may further compound CVD risk. Importantly, people living with HIV who also identify as LGBTQ experience a significant amount of stress, including difficulties finding a job or maintaining employment due to societal stigma and marginalization of HIV and their LGBTQ identities (Smit et al., 2012). In particular, LGBT PoC experience harassment, discrimination, and hostility in work settings (Bostwick, Boyd, Hughes, West, & McCabe, 2014). These findings extend to other countries, as found in an examination of LGBTQ workers in Spain, where perceived discrimination, functioning as a psychosocial stressor, was associated with work-related stress, depression, and risk of developing other mental health disorders (Moya & Moya-Garofano, 2020). More recently, there has been increased attention on the impact of intersectional discrimination for HIV (Marcellin, Bauer, & Scheim, 2013) and CVD (Caceres et al., 2020) in racial/ethnic LGBTQ. Hence, there is a need to know how intersectional discrimination impacts comorbid HIV and CVD risk, particularly for LGBTQ PoC.

Intersectional Discrimination

In general, society has difficulty with understanding and interacting with people who hold multiple stigmatized identities, namely LGBT PoC. As a result, social interactions are a source of stress for racial/ethnic LGBTQ. When someone is treated differently due to their sexual orientation and racial/ethnic identities, this is referred to as *intersectional discrimination*. The concept of intersectional discrimination has origins in the writings of Black feminists and critical race theorists of the 1970s and 1980s, in the context of Black women being discriminated against based on their racial/ethnic background and sex (Cho, Crenshaw, & McCall, 2013). Since then, this concept has expanded to include the oppression, namely anti-queer hate crimes and racist experiences, that LGBTQ PoC face from society (Meyer, 2008).

Intersectional Discrimination and HIV Risk for Racial/ Ethnic LGBTQ

Intersectional discrimination can have an insidious impact on risk for HIV among LGBTQ PoC. For example, English et al. (2020) show that discrimination prevalence by police and law enforcement toward Black gay and bisexual men was high, with 43% of the sample reporting these experiences. The investigators also indicated that incarceration history was positively linked to discrimination by police and law enforcement officers, which was associated with greater HIV risk. Moreover, despite the fact that women are seen as low risk for HIV infection, social, political, and economic level discrimination can contribute to LGB women's HIV risk development (Logie, James, Tharao, & Loutfy, 2012). Structural factors such as racial segregation, violence, discrimination enacted by health-care professionals and incompetent treatment by doctors raise the risk for HIV infection in African and Caribbean LGB women, which in turn increases allostatic load, that is, wear and tear of the body (Logie et al., 2012). Additionally, in a sample of transgender PoC in Canada, experiences of transphobia and racism interacted and produced greater odds of HIV-related risk (Marcellin, Bauer, & Scheim, 2013). Thus, these investigations indicate social, structural, and political forces play a significant role in HIV risk for LGBTQ PoC by enacting and perpetuating intersectional discrimination toward these communities.

Intersectional Discrimination and CVD Risk for SGMs of Color

Minority stress theory indicates that stress may lead to poor cardiovascular health outcomes through compromised psychological and physiological stress response pathways (Hatzenbuehler, Nolen-Hoeksema, & Dovidio, 2009). Data indicate that heterosexist harassment, rejection, and discrimination toward sexual minority adults are associated with CVD risk (Hatzenbuehler et al., 2009). A recent study also found minority stress was associated with greater likelihood of current smoking in Black and Latino LGB persons (Gordon et al., 2020). Moreover, data indicate that CVD RFs in Sexual Minority Women of Color are significantly greater than in White heterosexual individuals (Caceres et al., 2020). Another study examined the intersection of sexual identity and race/ethnicity effect on cardiometabolic RFs in Sexual Minority Women. The intersectional analyses found that Black lesbian and bisexual women are more likely to be obese and have higher rates of hypertension compared to White lesbian and bisexual women (Caceres, Veldhuis & Hughes, 2019). Results from this study suggest intersectional discrimination is associated with increased CVD risk among LGBTQ PoC, which may be reflective of increased allostatic load.

Intersectional Discrimination and Comorbid HIV and CVD Risk for LGBTQ PoC

Broadly, the effects of intersectional discrimination on HIV and CVD suggest that experience of sexual orientation/gender identity–based discrimination and racism are cumulative, which may lead to increased allostatic load, that is, wear and tear on the body. Currently, there are no studies that examine the long-term effects of intersectional discrimination on the comorbidity of HIV and CVD risk in LGBT PoC over time. However, Rich et al. (2020) have started a longitudinal study that aims to measure the associations of intersectional stigma and chronic stress in Black and Latina transgender women living with HIV. In particular, a focus of this study is to document the pathways linking chronic stress to HIV comorbidities, including CVD risk (Rich et al., 2020). This is a timely study, as it will address gaps in research on HIV comorbidities (CVDs in particular) among racial/ethnic gender-diverse PLWH.

CONCLUSION AND FUTURE RESEARCH

In sum, it is vital to examine the comorbidity of HIV and CVD in SGMs of color (SGMoC), as these communities are at high risk of developing comorbid HIV and CVDs. Regrettably, the literature for these communities remains underdeveloped, with clearly unmet needs. It may be that comorbid HIV and CVD risk are interrelated with mental health, behavior, and social/structural stigma, which result or further perpetuate instances of intersectional discrimination, unemployment, stigma, and harassment faced by racial/ethnic PoC. Therefore, the next wave of this emerging research must acknowledge the complex comorbidity of HIV and CVDs and incorporate the unique intersectional discrimination experiences that racial/ethnic LGBTQ people face from society.

REFERENCES

Barnes, R. P., Lacson, J. C. A., & Bahrami, H. (2017). HIV infection and risk of cardiovascular diseases beyond coronary artery disease. *Current Atherosclerosis Reports, 19*(5), 20. https://doi.org/10.1007/s11883-017-0652-3

Biglu, M. H., Ghavami, M., & Biglu, S. (2016). Cardiovascular diseases in the mirror of science. *Journal of Cardiovascular and Thoracic Research, 8*(4), 158–163. https://doi.org/10.15171/jcvtr.2016.32

Bostwick, W. B., Boyd, C. J., Hughes, T. L., West, B. T., & McCabe, S. E. (2014). Discrimination and mental health among lesbian, gay, and bisexual adults in the United States. *The American Journal of Orthopsychiatry, 84*(1), 35–45. https://doi.org/10.1037/h0098851

Caceres, B. A., Ancheta, A. J., Dorsen, C., Newlin-Lew, K., Edmondson, D., & Hughes, T. L. (2020). A population-based study of the intersection of sexual identity and race/ethnicity on physiological risk factors for CVD among US adults (ages 18–59). *Ethnicity & Health, 11*, 1–22. https://doi.org/10.1080/13557858.2020.1740174.

Caceres, B. A., Brody, A., Luscombe, R. E., Primiano, J. E., Marusca, P., Sitts, E. M., ... Chyun, D. (2017). A systematic review of cardiovascular disease in sexual minorities. *American Journal of Public Health, 107*(4), e13–e21. https://doi.org/10.2105/AJPH.2016.303630

Caceres, B. A., Veldhuis, C. B., & Hughes, T. L. (2019). Racial/ethnic differences in cardiometabolic risk in a community sample of sexual minority women. *Health Equity, 3*(1), 350–359. https://doi.org/10.1089/heq.2019.0024

Center for Disease Control and Prevention. (2017). *HIV and gay and bisexual men.* Retrieved from: https://www.cdc.gov/hiv/group/msm/index.html

Cho, S., Crenshaw, K. W., & McCall, L. (2013). Toward a field of intersectionality studies: Theory, applications, and praxis. *Signs: Journal of Women in Culture and Society, 38*(4), 785–810. https://www.jstor.org/stable/10.1086/669608

Chow, F. C., Regan, S., Feske, S., Meigs, J. B., Grinspoon, S. K., & Triant, V. A. (2012). Comparison of ischemic stroke incidence in HIV-infected and non-HIV-infected patients in a US health care system. *Journal of Acquired Immune Deficiency Syndromes, 60*(4), 351–358. https://doi.org/10.1097/QAI.0b013e31825c7f24

English, D., Carter, J. A., Forbes, N., Bowleg, L., Malebranche, D. J., Talan, A. J., & Rendina, H. J. (2020). Intersectional discrimination, positive feelings, and health indicators among Black sexual minority men. *Health Psychology, 39*(3), 220–229. https://doi.org/10.1037/hea0000837

Feinstein, B. A., Dyar, C., Li, D. H., Whitton, S. W., Newcomb, M. E., & Mustanski, B. (2019). The longitudinal associations between outness and health outcomes among gay/lesbian versus bisexual emerging adults. *Archives of Sexual Behavior, 48*(4), 1111–1126. https://doi.org/10.1007/s10508-018-1221-8

Freiberg, M. S., Chang, C. C., Kuller, L. H., Skanderson, M., Lowy, E., Kraemer, …, Justice, A. C. (2013). HIV infection and the risk of acute myocardial infarction. *JAMA Internal Medicine, 173*(8), 614–622. https://doi.org/10.1001/jamainternmed.2013.3728.

Gamble-George, J. C., Longenecker, C. T., Webel, A. R., Au, D. H., Brown, A. F., Bosworth, H., … & Implementation Research to Develop Interventions for People Living with HIV (PRECluDE) Consortium (2020). ImPlementation REsearCh to DEvelop Interventions for People Living with HIV (the PRECluDE consortium): Combatting chronic disease comorbidities in HIV populations through implementation research. *Progress in Cardiovascular Diseases, 63*(2), 79–91. https://doi.org/10.1016/j.pcad.2020.03.006

Gerbi, G. B., Habtemariam, T., Robnett, V., Nganwa, D., & Tameru, B. (2012). Psychosocial factors as predictors of HIV/AIDS risky behaviors among people living with HIV/AIDS. *Journal of AIDS and HIV Research (Online), 4*(1), 8–16. https://doi.org/10.5897/jahr11.057

Gordon, A. R., Fish, J. N., Kiekens, W. J., Lightfoot, M., Frost, D. M., & Russell, S. T. (2020). Cigarette smoking and minority stress across age cohorts in a national sample of sexual minorities: Results from the Generations Study. *Annals of Behavioral Medicine*, kaaa079. https://doi.org/10.1093/abm/kaaa079.

Grinspoon, S. K., Douglas, P. S., Hoffmann, U., & Ribaudo, H. J. (2020). Leveraging a landmark trial of primary cardiovascular disease prevention in human immunodeficiency virus: Introduction from the REPRIEVE coprincipal investigators. *The Journal of Infectious Diseases, 222*(Suppl. 1), S1–S7. https://doi.org/10.1093/infdis/jiaa098

Hanna, D. B., Guo, M., Bůžková, P., Miller, T. L., Post, W. S., Stein, J. H., … Shikuma, C. M. (2016). HIV infection and carotid artery intima-media thickness: Pooled analyses across 5 cohorts of the NHLBI HIV-CVD collaborative. *Clinical Infectious Diseases, 63*(2), 249–256. https://doi.org/10.1093/cid/ciw261

Hatzenbuehler, M. L., Nolen-Hoeksema, S., & Dovidio, J. (2009). How does stigma 'get under the skin?:' The mediating role of emotion regulation. *Psychological Science, 20*(10), 1282–1289. https://doi.org/10.1111/j.1467-9280.2009.02441.x

Hsue, P. Y., & Waters, D. D. (2018). Time to recognize HIV infection as a major cardiovascular risk factor. *Circulation, 138*(11), 1113–1115. https://doi.org/10.1161/CIRCULATIONAHA.118.036211

Kaplan, R. C., Hanna, D. B., & Kizer, J. R. (2016). Recent insights into cardiovascular disease (CVD) risk among HIV-infected adults. *Current HIV/AIDS Reports, 13*(1), 44–52. https://doi.org/10.1007/s11904-016-0301-4

Levy, M. E., Anastos, K., Levine, S. R., Plankey, M., Castel, A. D., Molock, S., …, & Weber, K. M. (2020). Depression and psychosocial stress are associated with subclinical carotid atherosclerosis among women living with HIV. *Journal of the American Heart Association, 9*(13), 1–15. https://doi.org/10.1161/JAHA.120.016425.

Logie, C. H., James, L., Tharao, W., & Loutfy, M. R. (2012). We don't exist': A qualitative study of marginalization experienced by HIV-positive lesbian, bisexual, queer and transgender women in Toronto, Canada. *Journal of International AIDS Society, 15*(3), 17392. https://doi.org/10.7448/IAS.15.2.17392

Mahungu, T. W., Rodger, A. J., & Johnson, M. A. (2009). HIV as a chronic disease. *Clinical Medicine, 9*(2), 125–128. https://doi.org/10.7861/clinmedicine.9-2-125

Marcellin, R. L., Bauer, G. R., & Scheim, A. I. (2013). Intersecting impacts of transphobia and racism on HIV risk among trans persons of colour in Ontario, Canada. *Ethnicity and Inequalities in Health and Social Care, 6*(4), 97–107. https://doi.org/10.1108/EIHSC-09-2013-0017

Meyer, D. (2008). Interpreting and experiencing anti-queer violence: Race, class, and gender differences among LGBT hate crime victims. *Race, Gender & Class, 15*(3/4), 262–282. https://www.jstor.org/stable/41674664

Morgan, E., D'Aquila, R., Carnethon, M. R., & Mustanski, B. (2019). Cardiovascular disease risk factors are elevated among a cohort of young sexual and gender minorities in Chicago. *Journal of Behavioral Medicine, 42*(6), 1073–1081. https://doi.org/10.1007/s10865-019-00038-z

Moya, M., & Moya-Garofano, A. (2020). Discrimination, work stress, and psychological well-being in LGBTI workers in Spain. *Psychosocial Intervention, 29*(2) https://doi.org/10.5093/pi2020a5

National Heart, Lung, and Blood Institute. (2020). *Coronary heart disease.* Retrieved from: https://www.nhlbi.nih.gov/health-topics/coronary-heart-disease

Nsagha, D. S., Assob, J. C. N., Njunda, A. L., Tanue, E. A., Kibu, O. D., Ayima, C. W., & Ngowe, M. N. (2015). Risk factors of cardiovascular diseases in HIV/AIDS patients on HAART. *The Open AIDS Journal, 9*, 51–59. https://doi.org/10.2174/1874613601509010051

Obry-Roguet, V., Brégigeon, S., Cano, C. E., Lions, C., Zaegel-Faucher, O., Laroche, H., ... & Poizot-Martin, I. (2018). Risk factors associated with over-weight and obesity in HIV-infected people: Aging, behavioral factors but not cART in a cross-sectional study. *Medicine, 97*(23). https://doi.org/10.1097/MD.0000000000010956

Rich, A. J., Williams, J., Malik, M., Wirtz, A., Reisner, S., DuBois, L. Z., ... Poteat, T. (2020). Biopsychosocial mechanisms linking gender minority stress to HIV comorbidities among Black and Latina transgender women (LITE Plus): Protocol for a mixed methods longitudinal study. *JMIR Research Protocols, 9*(4), e17076. https://doi.org/10.2196/17076

Saves, M., Chene, G., Ducimetiere, P., Leport, C., Le Moal, G., Amouyel, P., ... Raffi, F. (2003). Risk factors for coronary heart disease in patients treated with human immunodeficiency virus infection compared with the general popula-tion. *Clinical Infectious Diseases, 37*(2), 292–298. https://doi.org/10.1086/375844

Smeaton, L. M., Kileel, E. M., Grinsztejn, B., Gardner, E. M., Starr, K., Murry, M. L., ... Madruga, J. V. (2020). Characteristics of REPRIEVE trial partici-pants identifying across the transgender spectrum. *The Journal of Infectious Diseases, 222*(Suppl. 1), S31–S40. https://doi.org/10.1093/infdis/jiaa213

Smit, M., Cassidy, R., & Cozzi-Lepri, A. (2017). Projections of non-communicable disease and health care costs among HIV-positive persons in Italy and the U.S.A.: A modeling study. *PLoS One, 12*(10), 1–12. https://doi.org/10.1371/journal.pone.0186638

Smit, P. J., Brady, M., Carter, M., Fernandes, R., Lamore, L., Meulbroek, M., ... Thompson, M. (2012). HIV-related stigma within communities of gay men: A literature review. *AIDS Care, 24*(4), 405–412. https://doi.org/10.108 0/09540121.2011.613910

So-Armah, K., & Freiberg, M. S. (2014). Cardiovascular disease risk in an aging HIV population: Not just a question of biology. *Current opinion in HIV and AIDS, 9*(4), 346–354. https://doi.org/10.1097/COH.0000000000000065

Stevens, L. M., Lynm, C., & Golub, R. M. (2012). JAMA patient page. HIV infection: The basics. *JAMA, 308*(4), 419–419. https://doi.org/10.1001/jama.2012.4079

Virani, S. S., Alonso, A., Benjamin, E. J., Bittencourt, M. S., Callaway, C. W., Carson, A. P., ..., & Djousse, L. (2020). Heart disease and stroke statis-tics—2020 update: A report from the American Heart Association. *Circulation*, E139–E596. https://doi.org/10.1161/CIR.0000000000000757.

World Health Organization. (2017). Cardiovascular diseases (CVDs). Retrieved from https://www.who.int/news-room/fact-sheets/detail/cardiovascular-diseases-(cvds).

PART III

LGBTQ PoC Brain Health

CHAPTER 7

Cerebrovascular Disease Risk Factor Burden in LGBTQ PoC

James J. García and Mia Kijak

Abstract Cerebrovascular diseases (namely stroke) are the second leading cause of disability and mortality worldwide. Data highlight prominent racial/ethnic disparities in stroke risk factors, which are the same as those for heart disease, and suggest that communities of color experience greater stroke burden compared to Whites. An emerging, yet mirroring, literature for LGBTQ people is slowly surfacing and indicates that LGBTQ communities are more likely to report having had a stroke. However, there are limited data on the bio-behavioral and psychosocial stroke risk factor burden for LGBTQ PoC. Drawing from minority stress theory (Meyer, *Bulletin, 129*, 674–697, 2003) and allostatic load, this chapter argues that the cumulative effects of minority stress compromise brain health for LGBTQ people, with the greatest potential stroke risk demonstrated for LGBTQ PoC.

J. J. García (✉)
Department of Psychology, School of Health and Community Well-Being, University of La Verne, La Verne, CA, USA
e-mail: JGarcia4@laverne.edu

M. Kijak
Department of Psychology, University of La Verne, La Verne, CA, USA

© The Author(s), under exclusive license to Springer Nature Switzerland AG 2021
J. J. García (ed.), *Heart, Brain and Mental Health Disparities for LGBTQ People of Color*,
https://doi.org/10.1007/978-3-030-70060-7_7

81

Keywords Stroke • Allostatic Load • Intersectional Discrimination

Cerebrovascular diseases (namely stroke) are the second leading cause of disability and mortality worldwide (Johnson, Onuma, Owolabi, & Sachdev, 2016). Data highlight prominent racial/ethnic disparities in stroke risk factors, the same as those for heart disease, and suggest that communities of color experience greater stroke burden compared to Whites (Virani et al., 2020). An emerging, yet mirroring, literature for LGBTQ people is slowly surfacing, and shows that LGBTQ communities are more likely to report having had a stroke (Fredriksen-Goldsen, Kim, Shui, & Bryan, 2017). However, there are limited data on the bio-behavioral and psychosocial stroke risk factor (RF) burden for LGBTQ people of color (PoC). Drawing from minority stress theory (Meyer, 2003) and allostatic load (McEwen, 1998), this chapter argues that the cumulative effects of minority stress compromise brain health for LGBTQ people (Correro & Nielson, 2020), with the greatest potiential stroke risk demonstrated for LGBTQ PoC.

STROKE BIO-BEHAVIORAL RISK FACTORS

Similar to cardiovascular diseases (CVDs), stroke risk is partly driven by risk factors (RFs) that increase stroke burden. These RFs are classified as modifiable and non-modifiable. Evidence on the most studied RFs for stroke is discussed in this section.

Evidence from the INTERSTROKE study of over 32 countries offers the most robust data on the impact of modifiable RFs and acute stroke (O'Donnell et al., 2016). For example, the INTERSTROKE study found that ten modifiable RFs account for approximately 90% of stroke risk. In particular, hypertension or high blood pressure (defined as 140 mmHg/90 mmHg or higher) was associated with a nearly threefold risk for ischemic or intracerebral hemorrhage, accounting for 34.6% of population attributable risk (PAR) for a stroke; this is higher than the PARs of waist-to-hip ratio (26.5%), smoking (18.9%), diet (18.8%), cardiac causes (6.7%), ratio of apolipoprotein B to A1 (6.7%), depression (5.2%), diabetes mellitus (5%), psychosocial stress (4.6%), alcohol intake (3.8%), and psychosocial stress (4.6%). This suggests blood pressure accounts for the highest stroke burden, as found in countries across the globe (O'Donnell et al., 2010).

In the United States, extensive data show a disproportionately higher stroke burden for communities of color, as documented by the most recent American Heart Association/American Stroke Association statistical update (Virani et al., 2020). Importantly, evidence indicates that chronic stress increases stroke risk, particularly for Latinx, as found by the Hispanic Community Health Study/Study of Latinos (HCHS/SOL; Gallo et al., 2014). Regarding LGBTQ people, a national survey involving older and deaf LGBTQ persons found significantly higher odds of a stroke (50%) for LGBTQ people compared to non-LGBTQ persons (Kushalnagar & Miller, 2019). Considering the heightened stroke burden for communities of color, in addition to the increased odds of a stroke for LGBTQ people, it is plausible that those who identify as racial/ethnic LGBTQ have the greatest risk for stroke. The following section will present broad LGBTQ modifiable cardiovascular-related bio-behavioral factors, explore stroke findings in Transgender and Gender-Non-Conforming (TGNC) communities, and highlight specific LGBTQ PoC data disaggregated by race/ethnicity when possible.

Traditional Stroke RF Burden Among Sexual Minorities

Much of what is known about traditional RF stroke burden for lesbian, gay, and bisexual persons come from nationally representative datasets. This section will review notable stroke RF burden findings for lesbian, gay, and bisexual persons, whereas data are presented later in the chapter is focused on the small literature on the stroke burden of racial/ethnic LGBTQ.

Of the limited literature that exists, Caceres et al. (2018) examined stroke RF burden in over 395,000 lesbian, gay, and bisexual people from the 2014–2016 Behavioral Risk Factor Surveillance System. Results suggest that gay and bisexual men report higher rates of smoking, mental distress, and lifetime depression, but lower rates of obesity compared to heterosexual men. In contrast, lesbian and bisexual women demonstrated higher current smoking rates, mental distress, lifetime depression, heavy drinking, obesity, and higher physical activity compared to heterosexual women. Importantly, bisexual women had higher rates of stroke compared to heterosexual peers. In an analysis of the NHANES 2001–2012 dataset, Caceres et al. (2018) found that lesbian and bisexual women were more likely to be obese and have glycosylated hemoglobin (HbA1c) levels consistent with pre-diabetes compared to heterosexual women. Worthy to note, lesbian and bisexual women did not have significant differences in objective measures of hypertension, total cholesterol, or clinical CVD events. Unsurprisingly, these recent stroke findings corroborate the systematic review of Caceres et al. (2017) explained earlier in the CVD chapter of this edited text, providing convergent data on the increased vascular RF burden for LGBTQ persons.

In another nationally representative dataset, the 2013–2014 National Health Interview Survey, Fredriksen-Goldsen et al. (2017) found that older lesbian and bisexual women had greater odds for a stroke. This finding provides empirical support to the theoretical review of cognitive decline in LGBTQ older adults by Correro and Nielson (2020), who detail pathways in the development of adverse brain health outcomes for older LGBTQ, including stroke. More specifically, Correro and Neilson propose that LGBTQ discrimination uniquely contributes to social inequities by limiting access to resources, which elevates RF burden (e.g., smoking, mental distress, low physical activity), thereby increasing stroke risk.

Regarding objective stroke RF burden, in an analysis of the 2001–2010 NHANES using the allostatic load framework, Mays, Juster, Williamson, Seeman, and Cochran (2018) examined allostatic load via objective biomarkers. They found that bisexual men had greater levels of glycosylated HbA1c and systolic blood pressure compared to heterosexual men. Gay men, however, demonstrated lower AL compared to heterosexual peers, whereas no significant differences were found for lesbian and bisexual women. As such, there is compelling evidence of demonstrably greater stroke RF burden for lesbian, gay, and bisexual persons. Yet, limited data exist on stroke RF burden for racial/ethnic sexual minorities.

Stroke RF Burden in Gender-Diverse People

Despite recent and developing interest in LGB stroke health, few studies have focused on stroke RF burden for gender-diverse people, namely Transgender and Gender-Non-Conforming (TGNC) persons. Often, TGNC individuals are scarcely represented in the scientific literature, resulting in further marginalization of these communities. To this end, the following section highlights data about TGNC persons as well as what is known about stroke RF burden for these communities.

Mirroring CVD findings, an analysis of the 2014–2017 BRFSS, comprised of 1373 transgender men, 570 transgender women, and 570 gender non-conforming persons, by Caceres, Jackman, Edmondson, and Bockting (2020) found that transgender men and women had greater rates of self-reported stroke and were more likely to be overweight compared to cisgender men and women. Using the 2014 waves of the BRFSS, Meyer, Brown, Herman, Reisner, and Bockting (2017) found that transgender people had greater odds of having diabetes compared to cisgender persons. Moreover, findings from the New York–based Project AFFIRM revealed that experiences of discrimination (as minority stress) were associated with higher rates of risky drinking, lower physical activity, but not tobacco use or BMI for TGNC individuals which are in line with other findings (Caceres, Jackman, Edmondson, and Bockting, 2019). To further illustrate the CVD of transgender people, an analysis of over 600 transgender persons by Kidd, Dolezal, and Bockting (2018) found that legal document gender marker change (i.e., changes in gender-related legal documentation) was associated with lower tobacco use for trans-feminine persons, whereas gender-affirming surgery was predictive of lower tobacco use for trans-masculine people. However, hormone use among trans men was not associated with decreased tobacco use; this is concerning, given that the use of masculinizing hormones and smoking is associated with increased risk for a CVD clinical event, including stroke (Streed et al., 2017). Of note, the data presented are not stratified by race/ethnicity. Thus, results shed light on the TGNC RF profile, but indicate further research is needed to clarify stroke RF burden for racial/ethnic TGNC people.

STROKE RF BURDEN AMONG LGBTQ POC

As demonstrated earlier, there is substantial evidence to suggest sexual and gender minorities (SGMs) experience increased stroke risk. However, the stroke risk burden among racial/ethnic SGMs remains under-researched. To this end, this section will focus on highlighting stroke risk burden for racial/ethnic LGBTQ individuals.

In racial/ethnic LGBTQ youth, an examination of the Youth Risk Behavior Surveillance dataset by Beach et al. (2019) found that racial/ethnic lesbian and bisexual youth (comprised of 25.5% Latinx, 16.6% Black, and 10.2% other LGBTQ) were one to two times more likely to be overweight or obese compared to White heterosexual students. Furthermore, all racial/ethnic gay and bisexual groups were at the greatest risk of not meeting physical activity guidelines compared to White heterosexual male counterparts (Beach et al., 2019). Moreover, in an adult sample of the National Health Interview Survey, Caceres, Turchioe, Pho, Koleck, Creber, and Bakken (2020) examined stroke awareness among racial/ethnic LGB individuals. They found Hispanic and Asian gay, lesbian, and bisexual persons had lower awareness of stroke symptoms compared to White heterosexual men and women. In terms of stroke risk factors, an analysis of over 7000 men who have sex with men (MSM), conducted by Hirshfield, Downing Jr, Horvath, Swartz, and Chiasson (2018) found that Black MSM had greater odds of hypertension compared to White MSM. In contrast, Trinh, Agénor, Austin, and Jackson (2017) found no differences in diabetes prevalence, obesity, hypertension, or stroke risk among Latinx and White MSM. In their analysis of the 2014–2015 waves of the National Health Interview Survey, they examined the prevalence of health behaviors known to increase risk for stroke. Their analysis found that Black lesbian and bisexual women (compared to Black heterosexual women) were more likely to report heavy drinking, whereas Black and Hispanic gay and bisexual men were more likely to be current alcohol drinkers compared to White heterosexual men. Increased stroke RF burden is corroborated by the 2001–2012 waves of the NHANES, where Caceres, Brody, Halkitis, Dorsen, and Chyun (2018) found that lesbian and bisexual women of all racial/ethnic groups had higher BMI than White heterosexual women; Black bisexual women had greater systolic blood pressure and HbA1c than White heterosexual counterparts; Black gay and bisexual men had greater HbA1c than White heterosexual men; and Latinx who identified as "not sure" for their sexual orientation had higher systolic blood pressure, HbA1c, and total cholesterol compared to White heterosexual counterparts. Taken together, there is an increased stroke RF burden for racial/ethnic SGMs.

Stroke Prevalence

Regarding prevalence of stroke, limited data show greater prevalence of stroke for racial/ethnic LGBTQ. For example, Caceres et al. (2018) analyzed the NHANES 2001–2012 dataset and found Black lesbian and bisexual women had over a threefold greater prevalence ratio of stroke compared to White heterosexual women. Increased risk is also evident for those who identify as transgender. To illustrate, in a sample of 223 transgender women of color (TWoC) who were HIV positive seeking services from a community-based organization comprised of 85.2% Black/African American, 11.7% Latinx, TWoC over the age of 35 reported having significantly more strokes compared to younger TWoC in the context of

HIV/AIDS (Swartz et al., 2019). Therefore, there are some data indicating increased prevalence of stroke among racial/ethnic LGBTQ.

INTERSECTIONAL DISCRIMINATION AND CVD RISK FOR LGBTQ PoC

Given that intersectional experiences of social marginalization may be detrimental to health, the notion that those who have multiple socially minoritized identities (i.e., LGBTQ PoC) likely experience disproportionate stroke burden compared to their White LGBTQ counterparts is reasonable. To illustrate the impact of this these stressors, a study on the effects of minority stress on cellular functioning with gay and bisexual men found that leukocyte gene pathways related to cardiovascular functioning were perturbed as a function of greater experiences of minority stress (Flentje et al., 2018). Moreover, emerging data with racial/ethnic communities indicate that lifetime experiences of discrimination are associated with white matter lesion volume or subclinical cerebrovascular disease among Blacks (Beatty Moody et al., 2019). In a recently published study, minority stress experienced by White, Black, and Latino LGB persons was associated with greater likelihood of current smoking across middle and older age cohorts, as found in data from the nationally representative sample of the Generations Study (Gordon et al., 2020). Perhaps intersectional discrimination—as a unique form of minority stress targeting racial/ethnic SGMs—is a pathway in the development of increased stroke burden for LGBTQ PoC.

Despite this reasonable conjecture, there has been only one study to date examining intersectional discrimination and stroke RF burden among LGBTQ PoC. Caceres, Ancheta, Dorsen, Newlin-Lew, Edmondson, and Hughes (2020) examined the association between discrimination and RFs among 601 lesbian and bisexual women of color. They found that Black lesbian and bisexual persons were more likely to be obese and Black lesbians were more likely to report a history of hypertension and diabetes. Importantly, the discrimination assessment used did not specify which identities were targeted or whether questions assessed blatant or subtle discrimination. Furthermore, this study relied on self-reported RFs and did not include gender minorities of color. Thus, intersectional discrimination may increase stroke risk factor burden for LGBTQ PoC, but this literature is in the early stages of development.

SUMMARY

Research on stroke risk burden for racial/ethnic LGBTQ is slowly emerging, yet there is evidence of increased stroke risk demonstrated for these communities. Much like the calls to action made by Rosendale and Albert (2020), large cohort studies examining stroke risk in racial/ethnic SGMs are imperative to the advancement of this research. Moreover, studies conducted on stroke risk in racial/ethnic LGBTQ should focus on documenting epidemiological trends and use the frameworks provided by the American Heart Association/American Stroke Association (e.g., "Life's Simple Seven"); this may help facilitate data comparisons between larger datasets, increase visibility of study findings on stroke risk for racial/ethnic LGBTQ, and provide consistency with national health initiatives to identify and reduce stroke burden (Lloyd-Jones et al., 2010), particularly for racial/ethnic (Kulshreshtha et al., 2013) and LGBTQ communities (American Heart Association, 2018).

As described throughout this chapter, a focus on biological/objective markers is missing, as most studies rely on national datasets that utilize self-report/subjective methods. Without the implementation of biological/objective markers, results may lead to an underestimation of stroke risk for SGM PoC. Moreover, there must be a disaggregation of stroke type in the literature (e.g., ischemic stroke, subarachnoid hemorrhage, intracerebral hemorrhage) in order to better understand stroke in racial/ethnic LGBTQ. Additionally, the significance of intersectional discrimination as a psychosocial stressor is overlooked, despite the established impact of racism on stroke risk for heterosexual communities of color. Importantly, future research must explore stroke care disparities for LGBTQ PoC, given that these disparities are well documented for racial/ethnic communities (Cruz-Flores et al., 2011). Lastly, although not explicitly addressed in this chapter, a focus on traditional stroke RF models (e.g., using Framingham Risk Factor scores) to examine the predictive power of estimating stroke events in LGBTQ PoC is much needed; this may prove to be of strong practical value to the clinical management of stroke risk for health-care providers who work with these communities.

REFERENCES

American Heart Association. (2018). *More attention should be paid to heart health of lesbian, gay, bisexual 1adults, study suggests.* Retrieved from https://www. heart.org/en/news/2018/10/18/more-attention-should-be-paid-to-heart-health-of-lesbian-gay-and-bisexual-adults-study-suggests

Beach, L. B., Turner, B. C., Han, Y., Felt, D., Marro, R., Feinstein, B. A., & Phillips, G. L. (2019). Sexual orientation disparities in cardiovascular risk factors differ by sex and race/ethnicity among high school aged youth. *Circulation, 139*(Suppl_1). https://doi.org/10.1161/circ.139.suppl_1.P140

Beatty Moody, D. L., Taylor, A. D., Leibel, D. K., Al-Najjar, E., Katzel, L. I., Davatzikos, C., ... Waldstein, S. R. (2019). Lifetime discrimination burden, racial discrimination, and subclinical cerebrovascular disease among African Americans. *Health Psychology, 38*(1), 63–74. https://doi.org/10.1037/hea0000638

Caceres, B. A., Ancheta, A. J., Dorsen, C., Newlin-Lew, K., Edmondson, D., & Hughes, T. L. (2020). A population-based study of the intersection of sexual identity and race/ethnicity on physiological risk factors for CVD among US adults (ages 18–59). *Ethnicity & Health*, 1–22. Published online ahead of print. https://doi.org/10.1080/13557858.2020.1740174

Caceres, B. A., Brody, A., Luscombe, R. E., Primiano, J. E., Marusca, P., Sitts, E. M., & Chyun, D. (2017). A systematic review of cardiovascular disease in sexual minorities. *American Journal of Public Health, 107*(4), e13–e21. https://doi.org/10.2105/AJPH.2016.303630

Caceres, B. A., Brody, A. A., Halkitis, P. N., Dorsen, C., Yu, G., & Chyun, D. A. (2018). Cardiovascular disease risk in sexual minority women (18-59 years old): Findings from the National Health and nutrition examination survey (2001-2012). *Women's Health Issues, 28*(4), 333–341. https://doi.org/10.1016/j.whi.2018.03.004

Caceres, B. A., Jackman, K., Edmondson, D., & Bockting, W. (2019). Minority stress, social support, and cardiovascular risk factors in transgender and gender nonconforming persons. *Circulation, 140*(Suppl_1), A10202–A10202. https://doi.org/10.1161/circ.140.suppl_1.10202

Caceres, B. A., Jackman, K. B., Edmondson, D., & Bockting, W. O. (2020). Assessing gender identity differences in cardiovascular disease in US adults: An analysis of data from the 2014–2017 BRFSS. *Journal of Behavioral Medicine, 43*(2), 329–338. https://doi.org/10.1007/s10865-019-00102-8

Caceres, B. A., Makarem, N., Hickey, K. T., & Hughes, T. L. (2019). Cardiovascular disease disparities in sexual minority adults: An examination of the behavioral risk factor surveillance system (2014-2016). *American Journal of Health Promotion, 33*(4), 576–585. https://doi.org/10.1177/0890117118810246

Caceres, B. A., Turchioe, M. R., Pho, A., Koleck, T. A., Creber, R. M., & Bakken, S. B. (2020). Sexual identity and racial/ethnic differences in awareness of heart attack and stroke symptoms: Findings from the National Health Interview Survey. *American Journal of Health Promotion.* Published online ahead of print. https://doi.org/10.1177/2F0890117120932471

Correro, A. N., & Nielson, K. A. (2020). A review of minority stress as a risk factor for cognitive decline in lesbian, gay, bisexual, and transgender (LGBT) elders. *Journal of Gay & Lesbian Mental Health, 24*(1), 2–19. https://doi.org/1 0.1080/19359705.2019.1644570

Cruz-Flores, S., Rabinstein, A., Biller, J., Elkind, M. S., Griffith, P., Gorelick, P. B., & Peterson, E. (2011). Racial-ethnic disparities in stroke care: The American experience, a statement for healthcare professionals from the American Heart Association/American Stroke Association. *Stroke, 42*(7), 2091–2116. https://doi.org/10.1161/STR.0b013e3182213e24

Flentje, A., Kober, K. M., Carrico, A. W., Neilands, T. B., Flowers, E., Heck, N. C., & Aouizerat, B. E. (2018). Minority stress and leukocyte gene expression in sexual minority men living with treated HIV infection. *Brain, Behavior, and Immunity, 70,* 335–345. https://doi.org/10.1016/j.bbi.2018.03.016

Fredriksen-Goldsen, K. I., Kim, H. J., Shui, C., & Bryan, A. E. (2017). Chronic health conditions and key health indicators among lesbian, gay, and bisexual older US adults, 2013–2014. *American Journal of Public Health, 107*(8), 1332–1338. https://doi.org/10.2105/AJPH.2017.303922

Gallo, L. C., Roesch, S. C., Fortmann, A. L., Carnethon, M. R., Peñedo, F. J., Perreira, K., … Sotres-Alvarez, D. (2014). Associations of chronic stress burden, perceived stress, and traumatic stress with cardiovascular disease prevalence and risk factors in the HCHS/SOL sociocultural ancillary study. *Psychosomatic Medicine, 76*(6), 468. https://doi.org/10.1097/PSY.0000000000000069

Gordon, A. R., Fish, J. N., Kiekens, W. J., Lightfoot, M., Frost, D. M., & Russell, S. T. (2020). Cigarette smoking and minority stress across age cohorts in a national sample of sexual minorities: Results from the generations study. *Annals of Behavioral Medicine,* kaaa079. https://doi.org/10.1093/abm/kaaa079

Hirshfield, S., Downing, M. J., Jr., Horvath, K. J., Swartz, J. A., & Chiasson, M. A. (2018). Adapting Andersen's behavioral model of health service use to examine risk factors for hypertension among US MSM. *American Journal of Men's Health, 12*(4), 788–797. https://doi.org/10.1177/1557988316644402

Johnson, W., Onuma, O., Owolabi, M., & Sachdev, S. (2016). Stroke: A global response is needed. *Bulletin of the World Health Organization, 94*(9), 634. https://doi.org/10.2471/BLT.16.181636

Kidd, J. D., Dolezal, C., & Bockting, W. O. (2018). The relationship between tobacco use and legal document gender-marker change, hormone use, and gender-affirming surgery in a United States sample of trans-feminine and trans-masculine individuals: Implications for cardiovascular health. *LGBT Health, 5*(7), 401–411. https://doi.org/10.1089/lgbt.2018.0103

Kulshreshtha, A., Vaccarino, V., Judd, S. E., Howard, V. J., McClellan, W. M., Muntner, P., … Cushman, M. (2013). Life's simple 7 and risk of incident stroke: The reasons for geographic and racial differences in stroke study. *Stroke, 44*(7), 1909–1914. https://doi.org/10.1161/STROKEAHA.111.000352

Kushalnagar, P., & Miller, C. A. (2019). Health disparities among mid-to-older deaf LGBTQ adults compared with mid-to-older deaf non-LGBTQ adults in the United States. *Health Equity, 3*(1), 541–547. https://doi.org/10.1089/heq.2019.0009

Lloyd-Jones, D. M., Hong, Y., Labarthe, D., Mozaffarian, D., Appel, L. J., Van Horn, L., … Arnett, D. K. (2010). Defining and setting national goals for cardiovascular health promotion and disease reduction: The American Heart Association's strategic impact goal through 2020 and beyond. *Circulation, 121*(4), 586–613. https://doi.org/10.1161/CIRCULATIONAHA.109.192703

Mays, V. M., Juster, R. P., Williamson, T. J., Seeman, T. E., & Cochran, S. D. (2018). Chronic physiologic effects of stress among lesbian, gay, and bisexual adults: Results from the National Health and nutrition examination survey. *Psychosomatic Medicine, 80*(6), 551. https://doi.org/10.1097/PSY.0000000000000600

McEwen, B. S. (1998). Stress, adaptation, and disease: Allostasis and allostatic load. *Annals of the New York Academy of Sciences, 840*(1), 33–44. https://doi.org/10.1111/j.1749-6632.1998.tb09546.x

Meyer, I. H. (2003). Prejudice, social stress, and mental health in lesbian, gay, and bisexual populations: Conceptual issues and research evidence. *Bulletin, 129*(5), 674–697. https://doi.org/10.1037/0033-2909.129.5.674

Meyer, I. H., Brown, T. N., Herman, J. L., Reisner, S. L., & Bockting, W. O. (2017). Demographic characteristics and health status of transgender adults in select US regions: Behavioral risk factor surveillance system, 2014. *American Journal of Public Health, 107*(4), 582–589. https://doi.org/10.2105/AJPH.2016.303648

O'Donnell, M. J., Chin, S. L., Rangarajan, S., Xavier, D., Liu, L., Zhang, H., … Lopez-Jaramillo, P. (2016). Global and regional effects of potentially modifiable risk factors associated with acute stroke in 32 countries (INTERSTROKE): A case-control study. *The Lancet, 388*(10046), 761–775. https://doi.org/10.1016/S0140-6736(16)30506-2

O'Donnell, M. J., Xavier, D., Liu, L., Zhang, H., Chin, S. L., Rao-Melacini, P., … Mondo, C. (2010). Risk factors for ischaemic and intracerebral haemorrhagic stroke in 22 countries (the INTERSTROKE study): A case-control study. *The Lancet, 376*(9735), 112–123. https://doi.org/10.1016/S0140-6736(16)30506-2

Rosendale, N., & Albert, M. A. (2020). The intersection of sexual orientation, gender identity, and race/ethnicity on cardiovascular health: A review of the literature and needed research. *Current Cardiovascular Risk Reports, 14*(10), 1–7. https://doi.org/10.1007/s12170-020-00651-7

Streed, C. G., Jr., Harfouch, O., Marvel, F., Blumenthal, R. S., Martin, S. S., & Mukherjee, M. (2017). Cardiovascular disease among transgender adults receiving hormone therapy: A narrative review. *Annals of Internal Medicine, 167*(4), 256–267. https://doi.org/10.7326/M17-0577

Swartz, J. A., Ducheny, K., Holloway, T., Stokes, L., Willis, S., & Kuhns, L. M. (2019). A latent class analysis of chronic health conditions among HIV-positive transgender women of color. *AIDS and Behavior, 1*(12). https://doi.org/10.1007/s10461-019-02543-3

Trinh, M. H., Agénor, M., Austin, S. B., & Jackson, C. L. (2017). Health and healthcare disparities among US women and men at the intersection of sexual orientation and race/ethnicity: A nationally representative cross-sectional study. *BMC Public Health, 17*(1), 964. https://doi.org/10.1186/s12889-017-4937-9

Virani, S. S., Alonso, A., Benjamin, E. J., Bittencourt, M. S., Callaway, C. W., Carson, A. P., ... Djousse, L. (2020). Heart disease and stroke statistics—2020 update: A report from the American Heart Association. *Circulation*, E139–E596. https://doi.org/10.1161/CIR.0000000000000757

CHAPTER 8

HIV and Brain Health in LGBTQ PoC

Stephen Ramos

Abstract Given increased attention to improving HIV immunological functioning, the past decade has now focused on the impact of HIV on brain health. Current knowledge indicates HIV replication leads to immunological activation and production of neurotoxic and neuroinflammatory viral proteins, ultimately compromising neuronal integrity. Though there is no cure for HIV, effective treatments have allowed people living with HIV (PLWH) to live a long and healthy life. Nonetheless, the impact of HIV on the brain of PLWH persists despite viral suppression. These neurocognitive impairments result from HIV infection, with continued viral replication in the brain despite highly active antiretroviral therapy. This chapter focuses on understanding the impact of HIV on brain health for racial/ethnic LGBTQ, older adult LGBTQ PoC, and centers the role of intersectional discrimination for these communities as a unique psychosocial process that is currently underexplored in the science.

S. Ramos (✉)
Department of Psychology, Illinois Institute of Technology, Chicago, IL, USA
e-mail: sramos2@hawk.iit.edu

J. J. García (ed.), *Heart, Brain and Mental Health Disparities for
LGBTQ People of Color,*
https://doi.org/10.1007/978-3-030-70060-7_8

93

Keywords HIV-Associated Neurocognitive Disorder (HAND) •
Intersectional Discrimination • HIV and Aging LGBTQ PoC

Given an increased attention to improving HIV immunological functioning, the past decade has now focused on the impact of HIV on brain
health. Brown's (2015) seminal work identified HIV crossing the blood–
brain barrier into the central nervous system (CNS), through monocytes
and lymphocytes, with persistent infection seen in the perivascular macro-
phages and microglia (Temereanca et al., 2020). Current knowledge indicates HIV replication leads to immunological activation and production of
neurotoxic and inflammatory viral proteins, ultimately compromising
neuronal integrity (Elbirt et al., 2015; Rumbaugh & Tyor, 2015). While
the exact pathophysiology of HIV within the brain is not yet fully under-
stood (Simioni et al., 2010), exposure to neurotoxins and inflammations
creates the possibility for a spectrum of cognitive, motor, and affective
disturbances.

Though there is no cure for HIV, effective medical treatments (i.e.,
highly active antiretroviral therapy [HAART]) have allowed people living
with HIV (PLWH) to live a long and healthy life. Nonetheless, the impact
of HIV on the brain of PLWH persists despite viral suppression (Simioni
et al., 2010). These neurocognitive impairments result from the HIV
infection itself, with continued viral replication in the brain despite
HAART initiation (Oliveira et al., 2017). Moreover, persistent immune
activation in the plasma and cerebrospinal fluid may result in neurocognitive decline even with viral suppression (Spudich et al., 2019). Despite
extensive research on HIV-associated neurocognitive disorder (HAND)
with racial/ethnic communities, namely Latinx and Black/African
Americans (Rivera Mindt et al., 2020), this issue is understudied among
the aging lesbian, gay, bisexual, transgender, or queer populations (Clark,
Zinman, & Bomba, 2016), with no studies focused on LGBTQ people of
color (PoC). Therefore, there is an urgent need to understand the impact
of HIV on brain health for racial/ethnic LGBTQ, given the disproportionate burden of HIV experienced by these communities (Miranda,
Fuentes, & Rivera Mindt, 2014; Poteat, Scheim, Xavier, Reisner, &
Baral, 2016).

HIV-ASSOCIATED NEUROCOGNITIVE DISORDER

Before exploring racial/ethnic LGBTQ risk for HIV-associated neurocognitive impairments, this section presents a review of what/where neurocognitive impairments results from HIV. In particular, HIV-associated neurocognitive complications occur within the basal ganglia and white mater, resulting in mental slowing, memory loss, difficulties in complex tasks of executive function, and motor disorders (McArthur et al., 2005). As a result, HAND develops, reflecting a spectrum of neurocognitive disturbances that include the following (Antinori et al., 2007):

- *Asymptomatic Neurocognitive Impairment:* mild degree of HAND, categorized by objectively impaired neuropsychological performance, but absence of functional impairments.
- *Mild Neurocognitive Disorder:* second degree of HAND, in which daily function is mildly impaired.
- *HIV-Associated Dementia*: most severe presentation of HAND, categorized as an inability to complete daily tasks independently.

HAART as a Game Changer, Yet Neurocognitive Effects Still Remain

The use of HAART has successfully extended the life expectancy of PLWH; however, this has also introduced secondary complications, namely neurocognitive impairments (Krause, 2020). Worthy to note that with HAART treatment, the neurological deficits that PLWH experience are less pronounced compared to untreated HIV-associated dementia (Kusdra, McGuire, & Pulliam, 2002). Yet, mild forms of HAND remain quite common among individuals receiving HAART (Heaton et al., 2010). Indeed, an estimated 60% of PLWH on HAART will experience some degree of HAND (Schouten, Cinque, Gisslen, Reiss, & Portegies, 2011). Though prevalence of HIV-associated dementia has decreased due to HAART (Heaton et al., 2010), the continued neuronal and neuropsychological impact from HIV, despite viral suppression, suggests a critical need to focus on promoting optimal neurological protection for those at highest risk, including LGBTQ PoC.

BIOBEHAVIORAL AND PSYCHOSOCIAL RISK

Accelerated neurocognitive aging in PLWH is likely a result of multiple factors including HIV pathogenesis, treatment, and other opportunistic conditions (Heaton et al., 2015). These factors are associated with poorer health, particularly for individuals who exist at the intersection of their socially marginalized identities. Ilan Meyer's minority stress theory (2003) suggests that individuals from socially stigmatized groups often experience chronically high levels of stress. Chronic exposure to stress itself is an established risk factor for poor brain health (Watson et al., 2019). For example, a comprehensive literature review found that LGBTQ elders experience a variety of stressors throughout their life span, including judgment, rejection, prejudices, and internalized homophobia (Correro & Nielson, 2020). Such experiences of stress raise cortisol levels, a known contributor to poor neurocognitive health (Juster, Russell, Almeida, & Picard, 2016). For LGBTQ PoC, this includes race-related stressors such as discrimination and structural racism (Comas-Díaz, Hall, & Neville, 2019; Ghabrial, 2017).

In addition to single instances of unfair treatment, multiple sources of discrimination increase risk for adverse mental health including depression (Vargas, Huey Jr, & Miranda, 2020), and this has been observed in Black sexual minority women (Calabrese, Meyer, Overstreet, Haile, & Hansen, 2015). However, integrative research investigating the brain health of LGBTQ PoC is relatively new; therefore, it becomes difficult to conceptualize these risks, particularly for LGBTQ PoC living with HIV (Christofferson, 2017). That is, LGBTQ PoC living with HIV experience intersectional stress associated with society's minoritization of their identities. Understanding these risks as multifaceted and intersectional stress for LGBTQ PoC living with HIV is vital. Yet, to date, no study has systematically examined such risks for brain health with LGBTQ PoC living with HIV. This suggests a potential overlap in research agendas between racial/ethnic LGBTQ, HIV, and brain health (see Fig. 8.1).

Comorbidities

In exploring HIV and brain health, comorbid health conditions experienced by living with HIV commonly emerge. More specifically, PLWH experience medical comorbidities that are typically seen as diseases of aging. For instance, PLWH are more likely to have type 2 diabetes

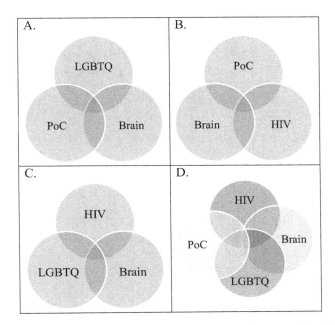

Fig. 8.1 Overlapping research agendas in the study of HIV and Brain health in LGBTQ PoC

compared to individuals without HIV (Galli et al., 2012). Additionally, some HIV medications carry the potential to increase the risk of type 2 diabetes in PLWH (HIVinfo, 2020). Epidemiological data indicate gay and bisexual men are more likely to report a lifetime diagnosis of diabetes than heterosexual counterparts (Beach, Elasy, & Gonzales, 2018) and it was well established that PoC have greater risk for diabetes (CDC, 2020b), and diabetes is associated with worsening cognitive health (Moheet, Mangia, & Seaquist, 2015). Similarly, hypertension dispropor-tionately affects racial/ethnic communities, with 54% of African Americans having a diagnosis of hypertension (CDC, 2020a), which can lead to dam-aged white matter that plays a central role in cognitive functioning (Iadecola et al., 2016).

In addition to bio-behavioral factors, depression is a known psychoso-cial factor in PLWH that is associated with worsening cognitive perfor-mance. Indeed, depression and HIV are expected to be the leading causes of disease burden by 2030 (Rubin & Maki, 2019). As it relates to brain functioning, depression is associated with increased impairment in executive functioning, delayed recall, verbal fluency, processing speed, and motor skill (Paolillo et al., 2020). Not surprisingly, a frequently cited meta-analysis reports that depression is associated with decreased CD4+ count and higher risk of mortality for PLWH (Leserman, 2008).

Discrimination as Psychosocial Risk for HIV and Brain Health

A comprehensive literature review found that HIV is disproportionately experienced by the First Peoples of Australia and Indigenous People of Canada, two groups with historical and ongoing experiences of discrimination (Rivera Mindt et al., 2020). These experiences of unfair treatment also extend to the health-care arena for LGBTQ PoC. As an example, Latina transgender women frequently report negative and discriminatory health-care experiences and providers responding negatively to their race, sexual orientation, and/or gender identity (Abreu et al., 2020; Howard et al., 2019). Moreover, men who have sex with men are commonly denied pre-exposure prophylaxis, an HIV preventative medication, though they represent the communities most affected by HIV (Furukawa et al., 2020). Contextually this is concerning, as Black gay and bisexual men face high levels of discrimination, which are associated with elevated HIV risk (English et al., 2020). Furthermore, studies with LGB people show that disclosing their sexual identity to healthcare professionals is a common phenomenon that spans across the globe (Pereira et al., 2019). These issues present as systemic barriers that prevent LGBTQ PoC from optimally utilizing health care for these communities due to experiences of intersectional marginalization.

The Role of Intersectional Discrimination as Trauma for LGBTQ PoC Living with HIV and Brain Health

Instances of intersectional discrimination (i.e., experiences of discrimination based on intersecting social identities and positions) including racism, sexism, and heterosexism (Holmes, Facemire, & DaFonseca, 2016) are related to HIV risk and comorbidities in Black and Latina transgender women (Rich et al., 2020). This intersectional oppression can be conceptualized as trauma (Holmes et al., 2016). Moreover, LGBTQ individuals are at higher likelihood of being abused within their families than their siblings, and individuals who are gender-non-conforming are often targets of hate crimes (Brown & Pantalone, 2011). Indeed, trauma is a known stress-related contributor to poorer neurocognition among PLWH. That is, the experience of traumatic events, financial hardship, and stress are more disproportionately experienced by PLWH than their seronegative counterparts. These combined experiences for PLWH are associated with poorer executive functioning, learning, working memory, and decline in activities of daily living (Watson et al., 2019).

Research also shows that individuals who identify as Latinx, Black, and Asian American experience higher risk for childhood physical and sexual abuse (Balsam, Molina, Beadnell, Simoni, & Walters, 2011). Importantly, childhood-related traumas, sexual abuse, and violence are commonly reported by PLWH, and these experiences have known consequences to the CNS such as structural and functional brain morphology and chronic exposure to stress-related hormones in the brain (Lupien, McEwen, Gunnar, & Heim, 2009; Sorrells, Caso, Munhoz, & Sapolsky, 2009; Watson et al., 2019). Together, these stressors pose high risks to neurocognitive health; however, science highlighting the role of intersectional discrimination as trauma in the context of brain health of LGBTQ PoC living with HIV is in its infancy (Rich et al., 2020).

Neurocognition in Aging LGBTQ POC Living with HIV and Brain Health

Neurocognitive decline in some domains (e.g., memory, processing speed) is a universal process of natural aging (Harada, Love, & Triebel, 2013). However, limited research investigating the experiences of LGBTQ older adults shows there is an increased risk for neurocognitive decline resulting from social marginalization in their proximal social environments (Fredriksen-Goldsen, Jen, Bryan, & Goldsen, 2018). In fact, a recent publication maps a preliminary model of health pathways for racial ethnic LGBTQ older adults, including intersectional threats of discrimination and ageism (Laganá, Balian, Nakhla, Zizumbo, & Greenberg, 2020). Moreover, findings from a recent study support some of the pathways of this model, with Black and Latino LGBTQ older adults reporting significantly greater subjective cognitive decline when compared to their non-PoC LGBTQ counterparts (Flatt et al., 2018). Importantly, subjective cognitive impairment may be representative of insidious cognitive decline, with PLWH experiencing a fivefold increase in subjective cognitive impairment compared to those without HIV (Sheppard, Woods, Massman, & Gilbert, 2019). Perhaps older LGBTQ PoC living with HIV are at an even greater risk of developing neurocognitive decline, given cognitive impairment is known to exist despite HIV viral suppression. Yet, this area of research is drastically under-investigated, as recent efforts document that the unique needs of LGBTQ PoC older adults are invisible in the literature (van Sluytman & Torres, 2014).

Undetectable = Untransmittable (U = U)

It is clear that HAART has significantly changed the impact of HIV, conferring protection against the progression of HIV to Acquired Immunodeficiency Syndrome. In addition, preventative approaches targeting those living with HIV have gained increased support, including HIV treatment as prevention and the Undetectable = Untransmittable (U = U) movement (Eisinger, Dieffenbach, & Fauci, 2019). More specifically, this movement has brought attention to HIV stigma, particularly for Black men who have sex with men (Meanley, Connochie, Bonett, Flores, & Bauermeister, 2019). However, as previously mentioned, neurocognitive impairments develop despite viral suppression (Heaton et al., 2010) and this may have greater impact for LGBTQ PoC. As demonstrated throughout this chapter, neurocognitive health is underemphasized in the healthcare needs of those who are virally suppressed and living with HIV. Thus, it would behoove researchers, clinicians, and community advocacy groups to underscore the importance of the neurocognitive impacts that still occur despite an undetectable viral load, with the explicit goal of promoting the long-term well-being of LGBTQ PoC living with HIV in today's society.

DISCUSSION

There are many potential factors related to neurocognitive health for LGBTQ PoC living with HIV. Dedicating individual chapters to each of these proponents of neurocognitive decline would only begin to do justice to this topic. However, without research to identify gaps in understanding, it becomes important to stress that these factors likely result in great risk for LGBTQ PoC living with HIV. That said, research investigating the neurocognitive health of LGBTQ PoC living with HIV is severely warranted.

REFERENCES

Abreu, R. L., Gonzalez, K. A., Mosley, D. V., Pulice-Farrow, L., Adam, A., & Duberli, F. (2020). "They feel empowered to discriminate against las chicas:" Latina transgender women's experiences navigating the healthcare system. *International Journal of Transgender Health*, 1–16. https://doi.org/10.108 0/26895269.2020.1767752

Antinori, A., Arendt, G., Becker, J. T., Brew, B. J., Byrd, D. A., Cherner, M., … Gisslen, M. (2007). Updated research nosology for HIV-associated neurocognitive disorders. *Neurology*, 69(18), 1789–1799. https://doi.org/10.1212/01. WNL.0000287431.88658.8b

Balsam, K. F., Molina, Y., Beadnell, B., Simoni, J., & Walters, K. (2011). Measuring multiple minority stress: The LGBT people of color microaggressions scale. *Cultural Diversity and Ethnic Minority Psychology*, 17(2), 163–174. https:// doi.org/10.1037/a0023244

Beach, L. B., Elasy, T. A., & Gonzales, G. (2018). Prevalence of self-reported diabetes by sexual orientation: Results from the 2014 behavioral risk factor surveillance system. *LGBT Health*, 5(2), 121–130. https://doi.org/10.1089/ lgbt.2017.0091

Brown, A. (2015). Understanding the MIND phenotype: Macrophage/microglia inflammation in neurocognitive disorders related to human immunodeficiency virus infection. *Clinical and Translational Medicine*, 4(1), 1–8. https://doi. org/10.1186/s40169-015-0049-2

Brown, L. S., & Pantalone, D. (2011). Lesbian, gay, bisexual, and transgender issues in trauma psychology: A topic comes out of the closet. *Traumatology*, 17(2), 1–3. https://doi.org/10.1177/1534765611417763

Calabrese, S. K., Meyer, I. H., Overstreet, N. M., Haile, R., & Hansen, N. B. (2015). Exploring discrimination and mental health disparities faced by black sexual minority women using a minority stress framework. *Psychology of Women Quarterly*, 39(3), 287–304. https://doi.org/10.1177/ 0361684314560730

Centers for Disease Control and Prevention (2020a). Estimated hypertension prevalence, treatment, and control among U.S. adults. Retrieved from https:// millionhearts.hhs.gov/data-reports/hypertension-prevalence-tables.html

Centers for Disease Control and Prevention. (2020b). *National Diabetes Statistics Report, 2020*. Atlanta, GA: Centers for Disease Control and Prevention, US Department of Health and Human Services. Retrieved from https://www.cdc. gov/diabetes/pdfs/data/statistics/national-diabetes-statistics-report.pdf

Christofferson, A. (2017). Intersectional approaches to equality research and data. Equality Challenge Unit. Retrieved from http://www.ecu.ac.uk/publications/intersectional-approaches-to-equality-research-and-data/

Clark, M., Zinman, H., & Bomba, E. (2016). Geriatric care and the LGBT older adult. In K. Eckstrand & J. Ehrenfeld (Eds.), *Lesbian, gay, bisexual, and transgender healthcare* (pp. 169–199). Cham: Springer. https://doi.org/10.1007/978-3-319-19752-4_12

Comas-Díaz, L., Hall, G. N., & Neville, H. A. (2019). Racial trauma: Theory, research, and healing: Introduction to the special issue. *American Psychologist, 74*(1), 1–5. https://doi.org/10.1037/amp0000442

Correro, A. N., & Nielson, K. A. (2020). A review of minority stress as a risk factor for cognitive decline in lesbian, gay, bisexual, and transgender (LGBT) elders. *Journal of Gay & Lesbian Mental Health, 24*(1), 2–19. https://doi.org/1 0.1080/19359705.2019.1644570

Eisinger, R. W., Dieffenbach, C. W., & Fauci, A. S. (2019). HIV viral load and transmissibility of HIV infection: Undetectable equals untransmittable. *JAMA, 321*(5), 451–452. https://doi.org/10.1001/jama.2018.21167

Elbirt, D., Mahlab-Guri, L., Bazalel-Rosenberg, S., Gill, H., Attali, M., & Asher, I. (2015). HIV-associated neurocognitive disorders (HAND). *Israel Medical Association Journal, 17*(1), 54–59.

English, D., Carter, J. A., Bowleg, L., Malebranche, D. J., Talan, A. J., & Rendina, H. J. (2020). Intersectional social control: The roles of incarceration and police discrimination in psychological and HIV-related outcomes for black sexual minority men. *Social Science & Medicine, 258*(113121). https://doi.org/10.1016/j.socscimed.2020.113121

Flatt, J. D., Johnson, J. K., Karpiak, S. E., Seidel, L., Larson, B., & Brennan-Ing, M. (2018). Correlates of subjective cognitive decline in lesbian, gay, bisexual, and transgender older adults. *Journal of Alzheimer's Disease, 64*(1), 91–102. https://doi.org/10.3233/JAD-171061

Fredriksen-Goldsen, K. I., Jen, S., Bryan, A. E., & Goldsen, J. (2018). Cognitive impairment, Alzheimer's disease, and other dementias in the lives of lesbian, gay, bisexual and transgender (LGBT) older adults and their caregivers: Needs and competencies. *Journal of Applied Gerontology, 37*(5), 545–569. https://doi.org/10.1177/0733464816672047

Furukawa, N. W., Maksut, J. L., Zlotorzynska, M., Sanchez, T. H., Smith, D. K., & Baral, S. D. (2020). Sexuality disclosure in U.S. gay, bisexual, and other men who have sex with men: Impact on healthcare-related stigmas and HIV pre-exposure prophylaxis denial. *American Journal of Preventive Medicine, 59*(2), e79–e87. https://doi.org/10.1016/j.amepre.2020.02.010

Galli, L., Salpietro, S., Pellicciotta, G., Galliani, A., Piatti, P., Hasson, H., ... Castagna, A. (2012). Risk of type 2 diabetes among HIV-infected and healthy subjects in Italy. *European Journal of Epidemiology, 27*(8), 657–665. https://doi.org/10.1007/s10654-012-9707-5

Ghabrial, M. A. (2017). "Trying to figure out where we belong:" narratives of racialized sexual minorities on community, identity, discrimination, and health. *Sexuality Research and Social Policy, 14*(1), 42–55. https://doi.org/10.1007/s13178-016-0229-x

Harada, C. N., Love, M. C. N., & Triebel, K. L. (2013). Normal cognitive aging. *Clinics in Geriatric Medicine, 29*(4), 737–752. https://doi.org/10.1016/j.cger.2013.07.002

Heaton, R. K., Clifford, D. B., Franklin, D. R., Woods, S. P., Ake, C., Vaida, F., ... Rivera-Mindt, M. (2010). HIV-associated neurocognitive disorders persist in the era of potent antiretroviral therapy: CHARTER study. *Neurology, 75*(23), 2087–2096. https://doi.org/10.1212/WNL.0b013e318200d727

Heaton, R. K., Franklin, D. R., Jr., Deutsch, R., Letendre, S., Ellis, R. J., Casaletto, K., ... Marcotte, T. D. (2015). Neurocognitive change in the era of HIV combination antiretroviral therapy: The longitudinal CHARTER study. *Clinical Infectious Diseases, 60*(3), 473–480. https://doi.org/10.1093/cid/ciu862

HIVinfo. (2020). Side effects of HIV medicines. Retrieved from https://aidsinfo.nih.gov/understanding-hiv-aids/fact-sheets/22/59/hiv-and-diabetes#:~:text=type%202%20diabetes.-,People%20with%20HIV%20are%20more%20likely%20to%20have%20type%202,diabetes%20in%20people%20with%20HIV

Holmes, S. C., Facemire, V. C., & DaFonseca, A. M. (2016). Expanding criterion a for posttraumatic stress disorder: Considering the deleterious impact of oppression. *Traumatology, 22*(4), 314–321. https://doi.org/10.1037/trm0000104

Howard, S. D., Lee, K. L., Nathan, A. G., Wenger, H. C., Chin, M. H., & Cook, S. C. (2019). Healthcare experiences of transgender people of color. *Journal of General Internal Medicine, 34*(10), 2068–2074. https://doi.org/10.1007/s11606-019-05179-0

Iadecola, C., Yaffe, K., Biller, J., Bratzke, L. C., Faraci, F. M., Gorelick, P. B., ... Saczynski, J. S. (2016). Impact of hypertension on cognitive function: A scientific statement from the American Heart Association. *Hypertension, 68*(6), e67–e94. https://doi.org/10.1161/hyp.0000000000000053

Juster, R. P., Russell, J. J., Almeida, D., & Picard, M. (2016). Allostatic load and comorbidities: A mitochondrial, epigenetic, and evolutionary perspective. *Development and Psychopathology, 28*(4pt1), 1117–1146. https://doi.org/10.1017/s0954579416000730

Krause, K. D. (2020). *Resilience as a buffer against negative health sequelae in older gay men living with HIV/AIDS: Implications for research and practice.* Unpublished doctoral dissertation, Rutgers The State University of New Jersey, School of Graduate Studies, New Jersey.

Kusdra, L., McGuire, D., & Pulliam, L. (2002). Changes in monocyte/macro-phage neurotoxicity in the era of HAART: Implications for HIV-associated dementia. *AIDS, 16*(1), 31–38. https://doi.org/10.1097/00002030-200201040-00005

Laganá, L., Balian, O. A., Nakhla, M. Z., Zizumbo, J., & Greenberg, S. (2020). A preliminary model of health regarding sexual and ethnic minority older adults. *Culture, Health & Sexuality,* 1–16. https://doi.org/10.1080/1369105 8.2019.1710566

Leserman, J. (2008). Role of depression, stress, and trauma in HIV disease pro-gression. *Psychosomatic Medicine, 70*(5), 539–545. https://doi.org/10.1097/PSY.0b013e3181777a5f

Lupien, S. J., McEwen, B. S., Gunnar, M. R., & Heim, C. (2009). Effects of stress throughout the lifespan on the brain, behaviour and cognition. *Nature Reviews Neuroscience, 10*(6), 434–445. https://doi.org/10.1038/nrn2639

McArthur, J. C., Brew, B. J., & Nath, A. (2005). Neurological complications of HIV infection. *The Lancet Neurology, 4*(9), 543–555. https://doi.org/10.1016/S1474-4422(05)70165-4

Meanley, S., Connochie, D., Bonett, S., Flores, D. D., & Bauermeister, J. A. (2019). Awareness and perceived accuracy of undetectable= Untransmittable: A cross-sectional analysis with implications for treatment as prevention among young men who have sex with men. *Sexually Transmitted Diseases, 46*(11), 733–736. https://doi.org/10.1097/olq.0000000000001048

Meyer, I. H. (2003). Prejudice, social stress, and mental health in lesbian, gay, and bisexual populations: Conceptual issues and research evidence. *Psychological Bulletin, 129*(5), 674–697. https://doi.org/10.1037/0033-2909.129.5.674

Miranda, C., Fuentes, A., & Rivera Mindt, M. (2014, January). Neurocognitive considerations in older ethnically-diverse HIV-seropositive adults. Retrieved from https://www.apa.org/pi/aids/resources/exchange/2014/01/ethnically-diverse

Moheet, A., Mangia, S., & Seaquist, E. R. (2015). Impact of diabetes on cognitive function and brain structure. *Annals of the New York Academy of Sciences, 1353*(1), 60–71. https://doi.org/10.1111/nyas.12807

Oliveira, M. F., Chaillon, A., Nakazawa, M., Vargas, M., Letendre, S. L., Strain, M. C., ... & Gianella, S. (2017). Early antiretroviral therapy is associated with lower HIV DNA molecular diversity and lower inflammation in cerebrospinal fluid but does not prevent the establishment of compartmentalized HIV DNA populations. *PLoS pathogens, 13*(1), e1006112. https://doi.org/10.1371/journal.ppat.1006112

Paolillo, E. W., Pasipanodya, E. C., Moore, R. C., Pence, B. W., Atkinson, J. H., Grelotti, D. J., ... Moore, D. J. (2020). Cumulative burden of depression and neurocognitive decline among persons with HIV: A longitudinal study. *Journal of Acquired Immune Deficiency Syndromes, 84*(3), 304–312. https://doi.org/10.1097/QAI.0000000000002346

Pereira, H., de Vries, B., Serzedelo, A., Serrano, J. P., Afonso, R. M., Esgalhado, G., & Monteiro, S. (2019). Growing older out of the closet: A descriptive study of older LGB persons living in Lisbon, Portugal. *The International Journal of Aging and Human Development, 88*(4), 422–439. https://doi. org/10.1177/0091415019836107

Poteat, T., Scheim, A., Xavier, J., Reisner, S., & Baral, S. (2016). Global epidemiology of HIV infection and related syndemics affecting transgender people. *Journal of Acquired Immune Deficiency Syndromes, 72*(Suppl 3), S210–S219. https://doi.org/10.1097/qai.0000000000001087

Rich, A.J., Williams, J., Malik, M., Wirtz, A., Reisner, S., DuBois, L.Z., Juster, R.P., Lesko, C.R., Davis, N., Althoff, K.N., Cannon, C., Mayer, K., Elliott, A., & Poteat, T. (2020). Biopsychosocial mechanisms linking gender minority stress to HIV comorbidities among black and latina transgender women (LITE Plus): Protocol for a mixed methods longitudinal study. *JMIR Research Protocols, 9*(4), e17076. https://doi.org/10.2196/17076

Rivera Mindt, M. G., Byrd, D. A., Morris, E. P., Tureson, K., Guzman, V., Summers, A. C., Crook, C., Savin, M. J., & Aghvinian, M. (2020). Cultural neuropsychology considerations in the diagnosis of HIV-Associated neurocognitive disorders. *Current Topics in Behavioral Neurosciences* (pp. 1-31). Springer. Advance online publication. https://doi.org/10.1007/7854_2019_121

Rubin, L. H., & Maki, P. M. (2019). HIV, depression, and cognitive impairment in the era of effective antiretroviral therapy. *Current HIV/AIDS Reports, 16*(1), 82–95. https://doi.org/10.1007/s11904-019-00421-0

Rumbaugh, J. A., & Tyor, W. (2015). HIV-associated neurocognitive disorders: Five new things. *Neurology: Clinical Practice, 5*(3), 224–231. https://doi. org/10.1212/CPJ.0000000000000117

Schouten, J., Cinque, P., Gisslen, M., Reiss, P., & Portegies, P. (2011). HIV-1 infection and cognitive impairment in the cART era: A review. *AIDS, 25*(5), 561–575. https://doi.org/10.1097/QAD.0b013e3283437f9a

Sheppard, D. P., Woods, S. P., Massman, P. J., & Gilbert, P. E. (2019). Frequency and correlates of subjective cognitive impairment in HIV disease. *AIDS and Behavior, 23*(3), 617–626. https://doi.org/10.1007/s10461-018-2297-9

Simioni, S., Cavassini, M., Annoni, J. M., Abraham, A. R., Bourquin, I., Schiffer, V., ... Du Pasquier, R. A. (2010). Cognitive dysfunction in HIV patients despite long-standing suppression of viremia. *AIDS, 24*(9), 1243–1250. https://doi.org/10.1097/QAD.0b013e3283354a7b

Sorrells, S. F., Caso, J. R., Munhoz, C. D., & Sapolsky, R. M. (2009). The stressed CNS: When glucocorticoids aggravate inflammation. *Neuron, 64*(1), 33–39. https://doi.org/10.1016/j.neuron.2009.09.032

Spudich, S., Robertson, K. R., Bosch, R. J., Gandhi, R. T., Cyktor, J. C., Mar, H., ... Godfrey, C. (2019). Persistent HIV-infected cells in cerebrospinal fluid are associated with poorer neurocognitive performance. *The Journal of Clinical Investigation, 129*(8), 3339–3346. https://doi.org/10.1172/jci127413

Temereanca, A., Ene, L., Rosca, A., Diaconu, C. C., Luca, A., Burlacu, R., … Ruta, S. (2020). Neurocognitive impairment in the combined antiretroviral therapy era in a Romanian cohort of young adults with chronic HIV infection. *AIDS Research and Human Retroviruses, 36*(5), 367–372. https://doi.org/10.1007/s13365-014-0275-1

van Sluytman, L. G., & Torres, D. (2014). Hidden or uninvited? A content analysis of elder LGBT of color literature in gerontology. *Journal of Gerontological Social Work, 57*(2–4), 130–160. https://doi.org/10.1080/0163437 2.2013.877551

Vargas, S. M., Huey, S. J., Jr., & Miranda, J. (2020). A critical review of current evidence on multiple types of discrimination and mental health. *American Journal of Orthopsychiatry, 90*(3), 374–390. https://doi.org/10.1037/ ort0000441

Watson, C. W. M., Sundermann, E. E., Hussain, M. A., Umlauf, A., Thames, A. D., Moore, R. C., … Moore, D. J. (2019). Effects of trauma, economic hardship, and stress on neurocognition and everyday function in HIV. *Health Psychology, 38*(1), 33–42. https://doi.org/10.1037/hea0000688

PART IV

LGBTQ PoC Mental Health

CHAPTER 9

Mental Health in LGBTQ PoC

Maleeha Abbas and James J. García

Abstract Social oppression (in the form of discrimination) takes a toll on the health of individuals. Indeed, extensive disparities in physical and mental health outcomes are evident for oppressed people, particularly sexual and gender and racial/ethnic communities. Despite their growing presence, racial/ethnic LGBTQ experience greater psychosocial stress from society's marginalization. Arguably, many of these experiences become salient in adolescence for racial/ethnic LGBTQ given development of these identities during this period. Therefore, adolescence represents a critical period in the development of mental health issues for LGBTQ PoC. This chapter draws from the minority stress theory as it relates to mental health disparities among racial/ethnic LGBTQ. Additionally, the chapter focuses on the importance of stigma and discrimination during

M. Abbas (✉)
Department of Psychology, University of La Verne, La Verne, CA, USA
e-mail: Maleeha.abbas@laverne.edu

J. J. García
Department of Psychology, School of Health and Community Well-Being, University of La Verne, La Verne, La Verne, CA, USA
e-mail: JGarcia4@laverne.edu

© The Author(s), under exclusive license to Springer Nature Switzerland AG 2021
J. J. García (ed.), *Heart, Brain and Mental Health Disparities for LGBTQ People of Color*,
https://doi.org/10.1007/978-3-030-70060-7_9

the critical period of adolescence, and how these experiences may lead to deterioration in mental health across the life span for LGBTQ PoC.

Keywords LGBTQ PoC Mental Health • Intersectional Discrimination • Substance Use • Adolescence

As discussed throughout the edited text thus far, social oppression (in the form of discrimination) takes a toll on the health of individuals. Indeed, extensive disparities in physical and mental health outcomes are evident for oppressed people, particularly sexual and gender minorities (SMGs; Herek & Garnets, 2007; Lewis, 2009; Meyer, 2003) and racial/ethnic communities (Williams & Mohammed, 2009; Williams & Williams-Morris, 2000). In the U.S., over nine million adults identify as Lesbian, Gay, Bisexual, Transgender, or Queer (LGBTQ; Meerwijk & Sevelius, 2017). Moreover, some data indicate there is an increase in the racial/ethnic LGBTQ population in the U.S., with Latinx being more likely to identify as LGBTQ (Newport, 2018).

Despite their growing presence, racial/ethnic LGBTQ have many negative experiences in the society. For example, literature documents that lifetime experiences of harassment, maltreatment, discrimination, and victimization for Black and Latino lesbian, gay and bisexual people is associated with poor mental health (Marshal et al., 2008). Moreover, work by Ghabrial and Ross (2018) indicates that only 7% of the research includes mental health outcomes for bisexual people of color (PoC). As a result of these compelling findings, it is essential to understand mental health problem experienced by racial/ethnic LGBTQ as a result of social marginalization in order to inform intervention efforts. This chapter will draw from the minority stress theory as it relates to mental health disparities among racial/ethnic LGBTQ. This chapter will focus on the importance of stigma and discrimination during the critical period of adolescence, and how these experiences may lead to deterioration in mental health across the life span for LGBTQ PoC.

Prevalence of Mental Health Issues

Mental health problems such as depression and anxiety are prevalent in LGBTQ communities. Research has found that bisexual people demonstrate higher rates of mental health issues comparison to lesbian and gay persons (Ross et al., 2017). Khan, Ilcisin, and Saxton (2017) found that, compared to White LGBT individuals, Black/African American and Latino/Hispanic LGBQ people reported higher suicide attempts.

Additionally, compared to heterosexual women of color and White lesbian and bisexual women, lesbian and bisexual women of color had the greatest risk of self-reported lifetime substance use. However, there is not enough quantitative research on prevalence of mental health in LGBTQ PoC, which leaves a big gap in the literature. Nevertheless, a recent qualitative study focused on the multiply marginalized experiences of LGBT PoC that include communities, identities, communication, and mental health (Ghabrial, 2017). Findings show that South Asian, African/Black American, Latino, Indo-Caribbean, and mixed-race LGBTQ experience disconnect from their communities, difficulties with personal relationships, and an inability to disclose sexual orientation to family. This, in turn, elicits stress and anxiety symptoms for LGBTQ PoC (Ghabrial, 2017). Similarly, LGBTQ older adults of color are often overlooked, and research has found that they suffer from isolation, fear of rejection, and intersectional discrimination, which adversely impact their mental health (van Sluytman & Torres, 2014). Therefore, there is a need for mental health research specifically representing LGBT PoC.

Minority Stress Theory

Broadly speaking, psychological and epidemiological research has investigated why the risk of mental health is greater for LGBTQ compared to their heterosexual counterparts. Findings from various disciplines highlight that the unique social marginalization experienced by LGBTQ functions as a chronic psychosocial stressor. Accordingly, stress experienced by LGBTQ people is referred to as *minority stress* (Meyer, 2003). This concept highlights the role of the social environment as a main source of stress for socially minoritized communities, which can create or lead to physical or mental health problems. Hence, social stress and adversity have a significant effect on the lives of people who belong from stigmatized social categories, including racial/ethnic LGBTQ.

According to the minority stress theory, when racial/ethnic LGBTQ people experience prejudice and discrimination related to racism, sexism, or homophobia, these experiences are mentally taxing (Meyer, 2003). In this view, racial/ethnic sexual and gender minorities (SGMs) must navigate the stress of living in heterosexist and racist environments (Meyer, 2003). Though not an explicit or central focus of this theory, the unique social experiences of racial/ethnic LGBTQ results from intersectional discrimination promoted and upheld by interlocking systems of oppression that shape their life experiences (Bowleg, 2013).

In a theoretical paper, Cyrus (2017) suggests that people who hold multiple minority statuses, including Black/African American, Asian, and Hispanic/Latinx LGBTQ, are exposed to significant stigmatization, discrimination, and experience greater fear of rejection when compared to their White LGBTQ counterparts. This model of multiple minority status for LGBTQ PoC proposes that the relationships between discrimination shape the social and emotional experiences of racial/ethnic LGBTQ. Moreover, racial/ethnic LGBTQ are negatively affected by cumulative discrimination and social exclusion, including racism from the broader LGBTQ community, and through the heterosexism and homophobia that exists within their racial/ethnic communities (Cyrus, 2017). The effects are further compounded by socioeconomic status, particularly for Black and Latinx LGB adults, and by difficulties with accessing culturally responsive and quality mental health care (Shangani, Gamarel, Ogunbajo, Cai, & Operario, 2020). Thus, examining factors like experiences of intersectional discrimination from society is vital to understanding LGBTQ PoC mental health.

INTERSECTIONAL DISCRIMINATION AND MENTAL HEALTH

Discrimination is a significant stressor that can lead to adverse psychological and emotional effects (Meyer, 2003). Indeed, LGBTQ PoC face unique experiences of intersectional discrimination that shapes their lived realities on a daily basis. Kimberlé Crenshaw coined the term intersectionality to explain the multidimensional experiences faced by Black women, including discrimination based on multiple social identities or positions, such as race, sexual orientation, and gender (Cho, Crenshaw, & McCall, 2013). To support the importance of this perspective, a recent study investigated discrimination, mental health, and suicidal ideation in lesbian, gay, bisexual, queer, and transgender adults, namely Black, Asian American, Latinx, and multiracial/multiethnic persons (Sutter & Perrin, 2016). The findings showed that LGBTQ-based discrimination had an indirect effect on suicidal ideation through mental health symptoms; however, racism had a direct impact on mental health symptoms. This could be an underlying factor that may explain why Black and Latinx LGB individuals are associated with increased risk of suicide attempts (O'Donnell, Meyer, & Schwartz, 2011). In addition, a recent analysis by Fattoracci, Revels-Macalinao, and Huynh (2020) found that intersectional discrimination performed better than heterosexism or racism alone in predicting mental health outcomes among LGB PoC. To further illustrate the unique predictive power of intersectional discrimination, research with Latinx gay, lesbian, bisexual, pansexual, and queer people shows that these communities have little support from their family members, struggle with traditional Latino gender role expectations, experience discrimination within the wider LGBT community because of their race, and face invisibility in the media. In particular, Noyola, Sánchez, and Cardemil (2020) found that intersectional discrimination experiences were linked to Mexican and Puerto Rican Latino cultural values, depression, and suicide ideation. More specifically, the intersectional experiences of LGBT and PoC predicted depression among individuals predicted higher depression symptoms and suicide ideation. However, identifying as LGBT or PoC on its own did not predict depression, highlighting the importance of intersectional experiences that are salient for Latinx LGBQ. Together, these data indicate that, above and beyond one instance of LGBTQ discrimination, intersectional discrimination has a substantial impact on LGBT PoC mental health.

In addition to blatant intersectional discrimination, LGBTQ PoC experience intersectional microaggressions, which are subtle hostile messages aimed at racial/ethnic or sexual gender-diverse individuals (Nadal, Whitman, Davis, Erazo, & Davidoff, 2016). Research shows that distinctive microaggressions exist for people who possess more than one stigmatized/minoritized identity. For example, when Black gay men hear comments like "Black gay people are so sassy," they may feel like their existence as a Black gay person is reduced to being a source of entertainment for others. Research by Fattoracci et al. (2020) examined whether intersectional microaggressions experienced by Black, Asian, Latinx, and Middle Eastern LGB people predicted adverse mental health outcomes. They hypothesized that intersectional racial/ethnic LGB microaggressions, that is, an intersectional approach, would be associated with worse mental health outcomes. The results showed that the intersectional approach was better at predicting greater anxiety over racial/ethnic or sexual orientation microaggressions alone. Thus, this highlights the overlapping nature of their existence as LGBTQ PoC at the intersection, with their unique experiences of discrimination best captured by using an intersectional lens.

Outside the U.S., transgender communities of color, particularly the *Hijras* of Pakistan, have gained visibility in countries where they are considered taboo. The *Hijras*, who identify as transgender women, experience high levels of discrimination in Pakistan, as they do not have access to fundamental rights such as health, education, and housing (Shah et al., 2018). These communities also report high levels of physical assault and institutional discrimination (Shah et al., 2018). Akhtar and Bilour (2020) found that despite high resilience, the *Hijras* sample reported low self-esteem, which is likely attributed to the chronic ostracization and marginalization of these communities in Pakistan (Grossman & D'Augelli, 2007). This ongoing maltreatment manifests in several ways. For example, transgender individuals are excluded and shunned by their families and friends, causing severe isolation (Grossman & D'Augelli, 2007). Moreover, research indicates *Hijras* who experience physical attacks and discrimination from employers, healthcare workers, and the general public show high levels of suicidality (Shah et al., 2018). Thus, the mental health of the *Hijras* is severely impacted as a result of intersectional discrimination from individuals, societies, and institutions.

SUBSTANCE USE, INTERSECTIONAL DISCRIMINATION, AND MENTAL HEALTH

Experiences of discrimination for LGBTQ PoC are also associated with substance use (McCabe, Bostwick, Hughes, West, & Boyd, 2010). For example, research with Black, Latinx and multiracial bisexual and gay men shows that the joint effects of racial discrimination and gay rejection are associated with emotion regulation difficulties, which in return predicts greater depression, anxiety, and heavy drinking (English, Rendina, & Parsons, 2018). Similarly, research with Latinx and African-American lesbian, queer, and bisexual women shows that intersectional discrimination is directly linked with alcohol-related outcomes (Cerezo & Ramirez, 2020). In particular, this study found that race and sexual orientation discrimination was a predictor of alcohol-related outcomes, with psychological distress mediating the relationship between alcohol use and intersectional stress. Together, these data suggest that intersectional discrimination adversely impacts the mental health of LGB PoC and increases risk for substance use.

Illicit drug use is another risky health behavior that is related to intersectional discrimination in LGBTQ PoC. Data indicate Black/African-African and Hispanic Latino LGBTQ individuals have high risk for illicit drug use (National Drug Intelligence Center, 2011). To explain this higher risk, Drazdowski et al. (2016) examined the cumulative effects of racism and sexual orientation discrimination in LGBTQ PoC. They found that greater instances of intersectional discrimination were associated with higher illicit drug use. These findings highlight the important role of intersectional discrimination on illicit drug use for LGBT PoC and illustrate that it is vital to develop psychosocial interventions targeting intersectional discrimination to reduce illicit drug use risk for racial/ethnic LGBTQ.

CRITICAL PERIOD OF ADOLESCENCE IN THE MENTAL HEALTH LGBTQ POC

Adolescence is a period of "storm and stress," often described as a time in critical development during which disregulation of behavior, emotions, and relationships are at their peak (Nichols & Good, 2004). The adolescent experience is quite unique for LGBTQ youth (Mustanski, Newcomb, & Garofalo, 2011). Indeed, a contemporary review found that the LGBTQ youth experience high isolation, rejection, phobia, marginalization, need for support, depression, self-harm, and severe suicidality (Wilson & Cariola, 2020). In a meta-analysis, sexual minority youth identifying as LGB reported suicidality three times as much compared to heterosexual youth (Marshal et al., 2011). A concerning finding in this meta-analysis is that LGBTQ youth of color showed significantly more suicidality than heterosexual youth (Marshal et al., 2011). Therefore, these issues are amplified for LGBTQ youth of color, who experience storm and stress differently from White LGBTQ youth, due to difficulties related to disclosure of their sexual orientation to their parents, friends, or family, while at the same time navigating shame and guilt from their racial/ethnic groups for identifying as LGBTQ (Aranda et al., 2015).

Research indicates that Black, Asian, and Latinx LGBTQ youth are at increased risk of domestic violence from adults, alcohol use, and trauma (Murphy & Hardaway, 2017). Importantly, the cumulative impact of experiences of discrimination negatively affects the mental health of LGBTQ PoC, resulting in a wear and tear of mental health that starts in adolescence. For example, studies have shown that mental health outcomes are worse for Black and Latinx lesbian, gay, bisexual, and queer youth (Toomey, Huynh, Jones, Lee, & Revels-Macalinao, 2017). Moreover, Black and Latinx LGBTQ youth experience significantly more mental health problems, like increased suicidal behaviors and hopelessness, compared to White LGBTQ youth (Russell, Sinclair, Poteat, & Koenig, 2012). Additionally, Black LGB youth report greater stressors that increase the likelihood of depression, anxiety, and suicide risk compared to Latinx LGB youth (Craig & McInroy, 2013). Thus, data indicate that LGBTQ PoC youth start experiencing mental health disorders from the adolescent period, and these negative experiences are cumulative over time, extending well into their young adult years and beyond.

These findings are corroborated in an international context. For example, a study in Japan examined suicidality and non-suicidal self-harm in those who identified as lesbian, gay, bisexual, and pansexual (DiStefano, 2008). The results showed behaviors of suicidality and non-suicidal self-harm are significantly associated with the homophobic environment of Japanese society. Moreover, suicidality and non-suicidal self-harm were significantly related to poor mental health, including greater symptoms of depression and anxiety.

CONCLUSION AND FUTURE RESEARCH

There are several things to focus on in the study of mental health disparities for LGBT PoC. First, it is essential to center intersectionality, as LGBTQ PoC experience societal marginalization from multiple sources. Second, it is important to examine within-group differences in mental health outcomes for LGBTQ PoC; that is, LGBTQ PoC should be disaggregated as groups and centered in research, as opposed to controlling for the effects of race/ethnicity in analyses, which neglects the rich narratives surrounding marginalization and exclusion form society for existing at the intersection of race/ethnicity and LGBTQ identities. Third, clinicians must routinely consider the intersectional effects of racial/ethnic and sexual/gender minority stress on mental health and substance use in LGBTQ PoC to provide culturally responsive treatment for these communities. Fourth, researchers and clinicians should examine the impact of intersectional stress faced by LGBTQ PoC during adolescence, as this period is vital for establishing mental health trajectories for these communities; doing so can lead to early prevention and treatment of mental health and substance use disorders among racial/ethnic LGBTQ across the life span. Lastly, a strengths-based approach to mental health resilience should also be explored, as preliminary evidence suggests the importance of a minority strengths approach to mental health in racial/ethnic LGBTQ (Perrin, Sutter, Trujillo, Henry, & Pugh, 2020).

REFERENCES

Akhtar, M., & Bilour, N. (2020). State of mental health among transgender individuals in Pakistan: Psychological resilience and self-esteem. *Community Mental Health Journal, 56,* 626–634. https://doi.org/10.1007/s10597-019-00522-5

Aranda, F., Matthews, A. K., Hughes, T. L., Muramatsu, N., Wilsnack, S. C., … Riley, B. B. (2015). Coming out in color: Racial/ethnic differences in the relationship between level of sexual identity disclosure and depression among lesbians. *Cultural Diversity and Ethnic Minority Psychology, 21*(2), 247–257. https://doi.org/10.1037/a0037644

Bowleg, L. (2013). "Once you've blended the cake, you can't take the parts back to the main ingredients:" black gay and bisexual men's descriptions and experiences of intersectionality. *Sex Roles, 68,* 754–767. https://doi.org/10.1007/s11199-012-0152-4

Cerezo, A., & Ramirez, A. (2020). Perceived discrimination, alcohol use disorder and alcohol-related problems in sexual minority women of color. *Journal of Social Service Research,* 1–14. https://doi.org/10.1080/01488376.2019.1710657

Cho, S., Crenshaw, K. W., & McCall, L. (2013). Toward a field of intersectionality studies: Theory, applications, and praxis. *Signs: Journal of Women in Culture and Society, 38*(4), 785–810. Retrieved from https://www.jstor.org/stable/10.1086/669608

Craig, S. L., & McInroy, L. (2013). The relationship of cumulative stressors, chronic illness and abuse to the self-reported suicide risk of black and Hispanic sexual minority youth. *Journal of Community Psychology, 41*(7), 783–798. https://doi.org/10.1002/jcop.21570

Cyrus, K. (2017). Multiple minorities as multiply marginalized: Applying the minority stress theory to LGBTQ people of color. *Journal of Gay and Lesbian Mental Health, 21*(3), 194–202. https://doi.org/10.1080/19359705.2017.1320739

DiStefano, A. S. (2008). Suicidality and self-harm among sexual minorities in Japan. *Qualitative Health Research, 18*(10), 1429–1441. https://doi.org/10.1177/1049732308322605

Drazdowski, T. K., Perrin, P. B., Trujillo, M., Sutter, M., Benotsch, E. G., & Snipes, D. J. (2016). Structural equation modeling of the effects of racism, LGBTQ discrimination, and internalized oppression on illicit drug use in LGBTQ people of color. *Drug and Alcohol Dependence, 159,* 255–262. https://doi.org/10.1016/j.drugalcdep.2015.12.029

English, D., Rendina, H., & Parsons, J. (2018). The effects of intersecting stigma: A longitudinal examination of minority stress, mental health, and substance use among black, Latino, and multiracial gay and bisexual men. *Psychology of Violence, 8*(6), 669–679. https://doi.org/10.1037/vio0000218

Fattoracci, E. S. M., Revels-Macalinao, M., & Huynh, Q.-L. (2020). Greater than the sum of racism and heterosexism: Intersectional microaggressions toward racial/ethnic and sexual minority group members. *Cultural Diversity and Ethnic Minority Psychology*. Advance online publication. https://doi.org/10.1037/cdp0000329.

Ghabrial, M. A. (2017). Trying to figure out where we belong: Narratives of racialized sexual minorities on community, identity, discrimination, and health. *Sexuality Research and Social Policy, 14*(1), 42–55. https://doi.org/10.1007/s13178-016-0229-x

Ghabrial, M. A., & Ross, L. E. (2018). Representation and erasure of bisexual people of color: A content analysis of quantitative bisexual mental health research. *Psychology of Sexual Orientation and Gender Diversity, 5*(2), 132–142. https://doi.org/10.1037/sgd0000286

Grossman, A. H., & D'Augelli, A. R. (2007). Transgender youth and life-threatening behaviors. *Suicide and Life-threatening Behavior, 37*(5), 527–537. https://doi.org/10.1521/suli.2007.37.5.527

Herek, G. M., & Garnets, L. D. (2007). Sexual orientation and mental health. *Annual Review of Clinical Psychology, 3*, 353–375. https://doi.org/10.1146/annurev.clinpsy.3.022806.091510

Khan, M., Ilcisin, M., & Saxton, K. (2017). Multifactorial discrimination as a fundamental cause of mental health inequities. *International Journal of Equity in Health, 16*(43), 1–12. https://doi.org/10.1186/s12939-017-0532-z

Lewis, N. M. (2009). Mental health in sexual minorities: Recent indicators, trends, and their relationships to place in North America and Europe. *Health & Place, 15*(4), 1029–1045. https://doi.org/10.1016/j.healthplace.2009.05.003

Marshal, M. P., Dietz, L. J., Friedman, M. S., Stall, R., Smith, H. A., McGinley, J., & Brent, D. A. (2011). Suicidality and depression disparities between sexual minority and heterosexual youth: A meta-analytic review. *Journal of Adolescent Health, 49*(2), 115–123. https://doi.org/10.1016/j.jadohealth.2011.02.005

Marshal, M. P., Friedman, M. S., Stall, R., King, K. M., Miles, J., Gold, M. A., ... Morse, J. Q. (2008). Sexual orientation and adolescent substance use: A meta-analysis and methodological review. *Addiction, 103*(4), 546–556. https://doi.org/10.1111/j.1360-0443.2008.02149.x

McCabe, S. E., Bostwick, W. B., Hughes, T. L., West, B. T., & Boyd, C. J. (2010). The relationship between discrimination and substance use disorders among lesbian, gay, and bisexual adults in the United States. *American Journal of Public Health, 100*(10), 1946–1952. https://doi.org/10.2105/AJPH.2009.163147

Meerwijk, E. L., & Sevelius, J. M. (2017). Transgender population size in the United States: A meta-regression of population-based probability samples. *American Journal of Public Health, 107*(2), e1–e8. https://doi.org/10.2105/AJPH.2016.303578

Meyer, I. H. (2003). Prejudice, social stress, and mental health in lesbian, gay, and bisexual populations: Conceptual issues and research evidence. *Psychological Bulletin, 129*(5), 674–697. https://doi.org/10.1037/0033-2909.129.5.674

Murphy, J., & Hardaway, R. (2017). LGBTQ adolescents of color: Considerations for working with youth and their families. *Journal of Gay and Lesbian Mental Health, 21*(3), 221–227. https://doi.org/10.1080/19359705.2017.1320741

Mustanski, B., Newcomb, M., & Garofalo, R. (2011). Mental health of lesbian, gay, and bisexual youth: A developmental resiliency perspective. *Journal of Gay & Lesbian Social Services, 23*(2), 204–225. https://doi.org/10.1080/1053872 0.2011.561474

Nadal, K. L., Whitman, C. N., Davis, L. S., Erazo, T., & Davidoff, K. C. (2016). Microaggressions toward lesbian, gay, bisexual, transgender, queer, and genderqueer people: A review of the literature. *The Journal of Sex Research, 53*, 4–5, 488–508. https://doi.org/10.1080/00224499.2016.1142495

National Drug Intelligence Center. (2011). *The economic impact of illicit drug use on American society.* Washington, DC: United States Department of Justice.

Newport, F. (2018). In U.S., estimate of LGBT population rises to 4.5%: Gallup. Retrieved from https://news.gallup.com/poll/234863/estimate-lgbt-population-rises.aspx

Nichols, S. L., & Good, T. L. (2004). *America's teenagers—myths and realities: Media images, schooling, and the social costs of careless indifference.* Routledge.

Noyola, N., Sánchez, M., & Cardemil, E. V. (2020). Minority stress and coping among sexual diverse Latinxs. *Journal of Latinx Psychology, 8*(1), 58–82. https://doi.org/10.1037/lat0000143

O'Donnell, S., Meyer, I., & Schwartz, S. (2011). Increased risk of suicide attempts among black and Latino lesbians, gay men, and bisexuals. *American Journal of Public Health, 101*(6), 1055–1059. https://doi.org/10.2105/AJPH.2010.300032

Perrin, P. B., Sutter, M. E., Trujillo, M. A., Henry, R. S., & Pugh, M., Jr. (2020). The minority strengths model: Development and initial path analytic validation in racially/ethnically diverse LGBTQ individuals. *Journal of Clinical Psychology, 76*(1), 118–136. https://doi.org/10.1002/jclp.22850

Ross, L. E., Salway, T., Tarasoff, L. A., MacKay, J. M., Hawkins, B. W., & Fehr, C. P. (2017). Prevalence of depression and anxiety among bisexual people compared to gay, lesbian, and heterosexual individuals: A systematic review and meta-analysis. *The Journal of Sex Research, 55*(4–5), 435–456. https://doi.org/10.1080/00224499.2017.1387755

Russell, S. T., Sinclair, K. O., Poteat, V. P., & Koenig, B. W. (2012). Adolescent health and harassment based on discriminatory bias. *American Journal of Public Health, 102*(3), 493–495. https://doi.org/10.2105/AJPH.2011.300430

Shah, H., Rashid, F., Atif, I., Hydrie, M. Z., Fawad, M., Muzaffar, H. Z., Rehman, A., Anjum, S., Mehroz, M. B., Haider, A., Hassan, A., & Shukar, H. (2018). Challenges faced by marginalized communities such as transgenders in Pakistan. The Pan African Medical Journal, 30, 96. https://doi.org/10.11604/pamj.2018.30.96.12818

Shangani, S., Gamarel, K. E., Ogunbajo, A., Cai, J., & Operario, D. (2020). Intersectional minority stress disparities among sexual minority adults in the USA: The role of race/ethnicity and socioeconomic status, *Culture. Health & Sexuality*, *22*(4), 398–412. https://doi.org/10.1080/1369105 8.2019.1604994

Sutter, M., & Perrin, P. B. (2016). Discrimination, mental health, and suicidal ideation among LGBTQ people of color. *Journal of Counseling Psychology*, *63*(1), 98–105. https://psycnet.apa.org/doi/10.1037/cou0000126

Toomey, R. B., Huynh, V. W., Jones, S. K., Lee, S., & Revels-Macalinao, M. (2017). Sexual minority youth of color: A content analysis and critical review of the literature. *Journal of Gay & Lesbian Mental Health, 21*(1), 3–31. https://doi.org/10.1080/19359705.2016.1217499

van Sluytman, L. G., & Torres, D. (2014). Hidden or uninvited? A content analysis of elder LGBT of color literature in gerontology. *Journal of Gerontological Social Work, 57*(2), 130–160. https://doi.org/10.1080/0163437 2.2013.877551

Williams, D. R., & Mohammed, S. A. (2009). Discrimination and racial disparities in health: Evidence and needed research. *Journal of Behavioral Medicine, 32*(1), 20–47. https://doi.org/10.1007/s10865-008-9185-0

Williams, D. R., & Williams-Morris, R. (2000). Racism and mental health: The African American experience. *Ethnicity & Health, 5*(3–4), 243–268. https://doi.org/10.1080/713667453

Wilson, C., & Cariola, L. A. (2020). LGBTQI+ youth and mental health: A systematic review of qualitative research. *Adolescent Research Review, 5*, 187–211. https://doi.org/10.1007/s40894-019-00118-w

CHAPTER 10

Psychosocial Risk and Resilience Factors in LGBTQ PoC Mental Health

David G. Zelaya, Caleb N. Chadwick,
and Cirleen DeBlaere

Abstract Sexual and gender minorities (SGMs) and racial/ethnic people are categorized as health disparity groups by the National Institute for Health. There has been a call to action for the field to examine the needs of individuals who hold SGM and racial/ethnic identities, including LGBTQ People of Color (PoC), who exist at the intersection of these

D. G. Zelaya (✉)
Department of Behavioral & Social Sciences, Brown University School of Public Health, Providence, RI, USA
e-mail: david_zelaya@brown.edu

C. N. Chadwick
Intraspectrum Counseling—Chicago, Chicago, IL, USA
e-mail: cchadwick@intraspectrum-chicago.com

C. DeBlaere
Counseling and Psychological Services, Georgia State University, Atlanta, GA, USA
e-mail: cdeblaere@gsu.edu

© The Author(s), under exclusive license to Springer Nature
Switzerland AG 2021
J. J. García (ed.), *Heart, Brain and Mental Health Disparities for LGBTQ People of Color*,
https://doi.org/10.1007/978-3-030-70060-7_10

121

identities. This task is not without challenges, as notable health disparities are evident in psychiatric symptomatology across the life span for LGBTQ PoC. This chapter will focus on identifying specific systematic factors and psychosocial risk and resilience perspectives to understand the mental health of these communities. In particular, the role of intersectional discrimination in mental health symptoms for LGBTQ PoC is highlighted.

Keywords Intersectionality • Intersectional discrimination • Resilience, Risk

Sexual and gender minorities (SGMs) and racial/ethnic people are categorized as health disparity groups by the National Institute for Health (NIH, 2020). There has been a call to action for the field to examine the needs of individuals who hold SGM and racial/ethnic identities, including Lesbian, Gay, Bisexual, Transgender, and Queer (LGBTQ) People of Color (PoC), who exist at the intersection of these identities. This task is not without challenges, as notable health disparities are evident in psychiatric symptomatology across the life span for LGBTQ PoC. Whereas the previous chapter focused broadly on mental health with racial/ethnic SGMs, this chapter will focus on identifying specific psychosocial risk and resilience perspectives for the mental health of these communities.

Research suggests that the onset of psychiatric problems among LGBTQ people, including LGBTQ PoC, begins in adolescence and continues into adulthood. For example, a 2020 National Survey of LGBTQ Youth mental health of over 40,000 participants, including 4000 Latinx, 1500 Black/African American, 1500 Asian/Pacific Islander, and 500 American Indian/Alaskan Native, revealed that 68% of the sample reported symptoms of generalized anxiety and 55% reported symptoms of depression within a two-week period, 60% reported sexual orientation or gender identity–based discrimination, and 48% reported incidents of self-harm within the past year (The Trevor Project, 2020). Additionally, Latinx LGB young adults who encounter family rejection are eight times more likely to attempt suicide and have close to a sixfold increased risk of developing depressive symptoms, compared to their counterparts who do not face— or have lower levels of—family rejection (Ryan, Huebner, Diaz, & Sanchez, 2009). Moreover, research the National Survey on Drug Use and Health shows that these mental health disparities persist across the life span, resulting in an overall greater risk for mental illness and increased risk for suicide (Substance Abuse and Mental Health Service Administration [SAMHSA], 2020). To build on these overarching data, focusing on the variability that exists within the LGBTQ population, is critical, with intersectionality and minority stress theory (MST) providing a helpful guide to understanding the lived experiences of racial/ethnic LGBTQ persons (Crenshaw, 1989; Meyer, 2003).

INTERSECTIONALITY AND MINORITY STRESS THEORIES

Intersectionality, as a theory, emerged from Black feminist and critical race theories to understand the unique discrimination experiences of Black women, inclusive of both racism and sexism, that resulted in systemic inequities (Crenshaw, 1989). However, intersectionality theory inherently acknowledges the nexus of multiple identities possessed by all marginalized people, including LGBTQ PoC, and the insidious experiences of stigmatization due to discrimination (Shin et al., 2017).

Historically, the scientific literature has understudied the experiences of individuals living at the "margins of the margins" in society, often examining LGBTQ PoC from heteronormative and White/Eurocentric lenses (Shin et al., 2017). This shortcoming is often attributed to the structural "intersectional invisibility" experienced by those holding multiple stigmatized identities (Moradi, DeBlaere, & Huang, 2010; Purdie-Vaughns & Eibach, 2008). For those studies that are inclusive of LGBTQ women of color (e.g., DeBlaere & Bertsch, 2013) and other LGBTQ persons of color (e.g., Velez, Polihronakis, Watson, & Cox, 2019), findings indicate that high levels of discrimination are consistently associated with greater psychological distress and decreased well-being. In the broader field, a content analysis of research with LGBTQ PoC (i.e., Black/African American, Latinx, Asian Americans, Native Hawaiians, Pacific Islanders, American Indians, Alaska Natives, and multiracial people) from 1969 to 2018 found that LGBTQ women of color (findings not disaggregated by race/ethnicity), particularly transgender and cisgender bisexual and lesbian women of color, continue to be underrepresented in the scientific literature (Barnett et al., 2019).

MST (Meyer, 2003) posits that these findings result from the unique stressors, above and beyond daily everyday stressors that individuals with marginalized identities experience. These distal (e.g., discrimination) and proximal (e.g., internalized oppression) stressors are associated with negative mental and physical health outcomes. Moreover, these stressors account for some of the observed disparities within LGBTQ populations. Extended to LGBTQ PoC, MST suggests that social marginalization produces stress related to membership in these communities and corresponding psychosocial experiences, including intersectional discrimination (Cyrus, 2017). Thus, intersectionality and MST inform our understanding of the unique experiences of LGBTQ PoC, as these perspectives acknowledge the complex social experiences of racial/ethnic LGBTQ. Therefore, the lived experiences of racial/ethnic LGBTQ will be discussed within the context of risk and resilience perspectives.

RISK FACTORS

To begin, the risk perspective argues that LGBTQ PoC exist as socially marginalized communities that experience greater psychological distress and reduced well-being compared to White LGBTQ or heterosexual PoC counterparts (Moradi, DeBlaere, & Huang, 2010). LGBTQ PoC encounter various risk factors at the personal and societal levels. The minority stress research literature has focused on conceptualizing psychosocial factors as a result of exposure to stress from identity-based discrimination, which increases risk for individual-level psychological processes (e.g., maladaptive coping; Hatzenbuehler, 2009). These risk factors interact with societal-level stigma and, in turn, affect individual psychological functioning. For example, the minority stress psychological mediation framework (PMF; Hatzenbuehler, 2009) suggests a number of mediating variables that potentially explain how adverse mental health outcomes develop for LGBTQ people. An established, yet growing, body of literature supports direct and indirect links between various forms of discrimination and psychiatric symptomatology for LGBTQ PoC, as found in a study that contained 33% Black/African American; 27.5% Asian/Asian American/Pacific Islander; 19% multiracial/multiethnic; 13% Latinx; 4.5% American-Indian/Native American; and 3% other (Sutter & Perrin, 2016). In the following section, we discuss how experiences of intersectional discrimination experienced by those who have socially minoritized identities create a unique risk milieu for the mental health of LGBTQ PoC.

Intersectional Discrimination

Increasingly, new measures are being developed to assess stressors associated with belonging to more than one socially stigmatized group and the links to mental health outcomes. Balsam, Molina, Beadnell, Simoni, and Walters (2011) developed the LGBTQ PoC Microaggressions Scale, finding that intersectional discrimination experiences (e.g., racism within the LGBTQ community) are associated with greater psychological distress. Additionally, Fattoracci, Revels-Macalinao, and Huynh (2020) developed an intersectional Microaggressions Scale for LGB PoC, which was found to better predict psychological distress, above and beyond measures of racial/ethnic and sexual minority microaggressions assessed separately. Analogous findings of the impact of intersectional discrimination as stress on mental health and social support were reported in a systematic review of 33 studies conducted with LGBTQ PoC in Canada (Sadika, Wiebe, Morrison, & Morrison, 2020). As it relates to proximal factors, internalized heterosexism in a study of LGBQ African Americans (Szymanski & Gupta, 2009) and sexual orientation concealment in a sample of LGB PoC (20% Latinx, 16% African American/Black, 8% Asian American/Pacific Islander, 5% multiracial; Moradi et al., 2010) demonstrate consistent and positive associations with mental health concerns, including maladaptive coping strategies (e.g., substance use) for LGBTQ PoC, namely Black and Asian/Pacific Islander (Drazdowski et al., 2016). Therefore, instances of intersectional discrimination functions as a risk factor, thereby influencing the mental health of LGBTQ PoC.

Psychological Factors

Minority stress research also focuses on risk from group-level psychological processes. These data emerge through Hatzenbuehler's (2009) psychological mediation framework in samples of LGBTQ PoC. For example, Ouch and Moradi (2019) found that affective expectation of stigma and emotion-focused coping self-efficacy mediated the relationship between discrimination and psychological distress in a sample of LGBQ PoC, including 33% African American/Black, 32% Asian/Asian American, 27% Latinx, 14% other such as Caribbean American, 8% American Indian/Native American, 5% Arab American/Middle Eastern/North African, and 3% Pacific Islander. Others have found support for rumination and social support processes as important mediators for the effects of stigma and mental health in samples of gay and bisexual Canadian men, where 14.2% were East/South East/South Asian, 11.3% mixed race, 6.7% Black, 5.8% Latinx, 1.9% Middle Easter/North African, and 0.9% Aboriginal (Schwartz, Stratton, & Hart, 2016). Thus, discrimination for LGBTQ PoC can be conceptualized within the broader context of societal-level oppression experienced by these communities.

Systemic Factors

There are also systemic factors salient to the day-to-day realities of LGBTQ PoC that increase risk for adverse mental health (Mayer et al., 2014). For example, one study focused on transgender PoC (i.e., eight Asian and Pacific Islander, six African American, six Latinx) found that these communities are likely to engage in sex work to pay rent and to afford gender-affirmative health care (Bith-Melander et al., 2010). Another study of transgender youth of color (84% Black and 13% Latinx) found they were more likely to have lower levels of educational attainment, increased housing insecurity, and more instances of transactional sex compared to cisgender young men who have sex with men (MSM) of color (Bauermeister, Goldenberg, Connochie, Jadwin-Cakmak, & Stephenson, 2016). Furthermore, once LGBTQ PoC access health care, they encounter discrimination from providers across various clinical settings such as mental health and substance use clinics, based on data from 852 biracial/multiracial, 290 Black, 217 Latinx, 137 Asian/Pacific Islander, 83 American Indian persons (Kattari, Walls, Whitfield, & Magruder, 2017). Together, these data underscore that LGBTQ PoC encounter systemic-level psychosocial risk.

An important observation in the literature is that the majority of studies examining systemic risk factors in LGBTQ PoC focus on White samples from the western hemisphere (e.g., Italy; Scandurra, Amodeo, Valerio, Bochicchio, & Frost, 2017) and this also extends to U.S. samples, which limits the generalizability of these findings to regions across the globe. Nonetheless, minority stress research is growing in prominence on an international scale. For example, Dunn, Gonzalez, Costa, Nardi, and Iantaffi (2014) provide evidence for the generalization of the minority stress model for a sample of predominantly gay and bisexual men from Brazil. Given the significant and increasingly prominent role of the risk perspective, scholars note the importance of utilizing a strengths-based approach to understanding the complex experiences of these groups (Vaughan et al., 2014).

Resilience Factors

In contrast to the risk model, the resilience perspective asserts that marginalized individuals possess unique strengths that confer a protective effect on their mental health (Moradi, DeBlaere, & Huang, 2010). Broadly, the resilience research literature for LGB people has found that individual hardiness, family strength, and community connectedness are promotive factors for resilience (Lira & Morais, 2017). Yet, the resiliency literature among LGBTQ PoC remains nascent and is largely comprised of qualitative studies. For example, one study, with a sample of transgender PoC (n = 6 African American/black, 3 Latino/Hispanic, 2 Multiracial), examined resilience after traumatic life events (e.g., hate crimes) and identified several themes such as pride, spirituality and hope, community support, and collective action as important factors (Singh & McKleroy, 2011). Moreover, Stone, Nimmons, Salcido, and Schnarrs (2020), in a sample of Black and Latinx and mostly LGBQ, found that mothers and "othermothers" (e.g., grandmothers) were strong models of resilience. In addition to individual-level resilience, group-level resilience such as resistance to oppression and psycho-political wellness is documented in the literature, specifically with Black Bisexual people (Mosley, Abreu, & Crowell, 2017).

Another promotive factor for resilience is intersectional pride, which qualitative and quantitative studies support as an important positive intersectional identity perspective (Ghabrial, 2017). For example, intersectional pride has emerged as a protective factor in the face of adverse experiences, including perceived racism, for racially/ethnically diverse LGBQ PoC samples (i.e., 3 East Asian, 2 Black/Afro-Caribbean, 2 Latinx, 2 multiracial, 1 South Asian, 1 Aboriginal; Ghabrial, 2017; 67 African American/Black, 33 Asian/Asian American/Pacific Islander, 25 Hispanic/Latina, 25 multiracial, 11 other race/ethnicities, 3 Native American/American Indian; DeBlaere & Bertsch, 2013). Similarly, connecting with communities relevant to their identities (e.g., communities of color and religious/spiritual communities) has been identified in Black lesbian women (Bowleg, Huang, Brooks, Black, & Burkholder, 2003), Latinx gay men (Gray, Mendelsohn, & Omoto, 2015), and racially/ethnically diverse LBTQ women (n = 372 Latinx, 171 Asian/Pacific Islander, 673 Black; Harris, Battle, Pastrana, & Daniels, 2015) as important sources of resilience. Furthermore, studies suggest social support acts as a protective factor for binegativity and psychiatric symptomatology in bisexual Latinx, Black, and American Indian/Indian people (Flanders, Shuler, Desnoyers, & VanKim, 2019). As a societal-level factor, civic engagement has been reported as a source of resilience in older Black lesbian women (Battle, Daniels, & Pastrana, 2015), Latinx gay and bisexual youth (Li, Thing, Galvan, Gonzalez, & Bluthenthal, 2017), as has self-advocacy or personal agency (i.e., power to enact change) in Black lesbian women (Bowleg et al., 2003) and transgender youth of color (sample included 6 African American/Black, 3 Chicana/Latino, 2 Asian American/Pacific Islander, 2 multiracial; Singh, 2013).

As demonstrated, research on resilience with racial/ethnic LGBTQ samples is steadily growing. Importantly, international findings are largely analogous to those from U.S. samples, despite the criminalization of LGBTQ identities in many countries (e.g., Russia; Wong, 2015). For example, connecting with critical communities and involvement in social justice activism were identified as themes in a sample of resilience in majority gay, lesbian, and bisexual persons from Nicaragua, Colombia, and 13 other countries (Almario, Riggle, Rostosky, & Alcalde, 2013). A qualitative study with civic engagement documented similar results to U.S. findings in a sample of majority gay and transgender men and women refugees and asylees from Africa, Middle East, and North America (Alessi, 2016) and with LGB people in China (Chong, Zhang, Mak, & Pang, 2015). Furthermore, in a small sample of migrant (e.g., Sub-Saharan Africa) bisexual PoC in Italy, narratives of self-acceptance and resistance were found to be a way to challenge societal-level discrimination (Castro & Carnassale, 2019).

CONCLUSION

LGBTQ PoC experience the effects of dynamic and serious risk factors, increasing their burden for negative mental health outcomes. Whether in the form of intersectional discrimination or systemic forms of oppression, these chronic risk factors are faced by communities with tremendous resourcefulness, despite adversity. Indeed, it is important to not discount this resourcefulness, as it manifests in powerful sources of resilience—all of which play a vital and protective role for LGBTQ PoC mental and physical health. Recent minority strengths frameworks have been developed, focusing on highlighting the empirical pathways involved in promoting resilience for racial/ethnic LGBTQ (Perrin, Sutter, Trujillo, Henry, & Pugh, 2020). In the spirit of working toward a more just society, restorative efforts must be comprehensive, focusing on identifying and mitigating the burden of substantial risk factors, while also leveraging sources of strength, power, and resilience demonstrated by racial/ethnic LGBTQ to promote their heart, brain, and mental health.

REFERENCES

Alessi, E. J. (2016). Resilience in sexual and gender minority forced migrants: A qualitative exploration. *Traumatology, 22*(3), 203–213. https://doi. org/10.1037/trm0000077

Almario, M., Riggle, E. D. B., Rostosky, S. S., & Alcalde, M. C. (2013). Positive themes in LGBT self-identities in Spanish-speaking countries. *International Perspectives in Psychology: Research, Practice, Consultation, 2*(1), 1–13. https:// doi.org/10.1037/a0031055

Balsam, K. F., Molina, Y., Beadnell, B., Simoni, J., & Walters, K. (2011). Measuring multiple minority stress: The LGBT people of color microaggressions scale. *Cultural Diversity and Ethnic Minority Psychology, 17*(2), 163–174. https:// doi.org/10.1037/a0023244

Barnett, A. P., del Río-González, A. M., Parchem, B., Pinho, V., Aguayo-Romero, R., Nakamura, N., ... Zea, M. C. (2019). Content analysis of psychological research with lesbian, gay, bisexual, and transgender people of color in the United States: 1969–2018. *American Psychologist, 74*(8), 898–911. https:// doi.org/10.1037/amp0000562.supp

Battle, J., Daniels, J., & Pastrana, A., Jr. (2015). Civic engagement, religion, and health: Older Black lesbians in the social justice sexuality (SJS) survey. *Women, Gender, and Families of Color, 3*(1), 19–35. https://doi.org/10.5406/ womgenfamcol.3.1.0019

Bauermeister, J. A., Goldenberg, T., Connochie, D., Jadwin-Cakmak, L., & Stephenson, R. (2016). Psychosocial disparities among racial/ethnic minority transgender young adults and young men who have sex with men living in Detroit. *Transgender Health, 1*(1), 279–290. https://doi.org/10.1089/ trgh.2016.0027

Bith-Melander, P., Sheoran, B., Sheth, L., Bermudez, C., Drone, J., Wood, W., & Schroeder, K. (2010). Understanding sociocultural and psychological factors affecting transgender people of color in San Francisco. *Journal of the Association of Nurses in AIDS Care, 21*(3), 207–220. https://doi.org/10.1016/j. jana.2010.01.008

Bowleg, L., Huang, J., Brooks, K., Black, A., & Burkholder, G. (2003). Triple jeopardy and beyond: Multiple minority stress and resilience among Black lesbians. *Journal of Lesbian Studies, 7*(4), 87–108. https://doi.org/10.1300/j155v07n04_06

Castro, A., & Carnassale, D. (2019). Loving more than one color: Bisexuals of color in Italy between stigma and resilience. *Journal of Bisexuality, 19*(2), 198–228. https://doi.org/10.1080/15299716.2019.1617548

Chong, E. S. K., Zhang, Y., Mak, W. W. S., & Pang, I. H. Y. (2015). Social media as social capital of LGB individuals in Hong Kong: Its relations with group membership, stigma, and mental well-being. *American Journal of Community Psychology, 55*(1–2), 228–238. https://doi.org/10.1007/s10464-014-9699-2

Crenshaw, K. (1989). Demarginalizing the intersection of race and sex: A black feminist critique of antidiscrimination doctrine, feminist theory and antiracist politics. *University of Chicago Legal Forum, 139*(1), 139–167. Retrieved from https://chicagounbound.uchicago.edu/uclf/vol1989/iss1/8

Cyrus, K. (2017). Multiple minorities as multiply marginalized: Applying the minority stress theory to LGBTQ people of color. *Journal of Gay & Lesbian Mental Health, 21*(3), 194–202. https://doi.org/10.1080/1935970 5.2017.1320739

DeBlaere, C., & Bertsch, K. N. (2013). Perceived sexist events and psychological distress of sexual minority women of color: The moderating role of womanism. *Psychology of Women Quarterly, 37*(2), 167–178. https://doi.org/10.1177/0361684312470436

Drazdowski, T. K., Perrin, P. B., Trujillo, M., Sutter, M., Benotsch, E. G., & Snipes, D. J. (2016). Structural equation modeling of the effects of racism, LGBTQ discrimination, and internalized oppression on illicit drug use in LGBTQ people of color. *Drug and Alcohol Dependence, 159*, 255–262. https://doi.org/10.1016/j.drugalcdep.2015.12.029

Dunn, T. L., Gonzalez, C. A., Costa, A. B., Nardi, H. C., & Iantaffi, A. (2014). Does the minority stress model generalize to a non-US sample? An examination of minority stress and resilience on depressive symptomatology among sexual minority men in two urban areas of Brazil. *Psychology of Sexual Orientation and Gender Diversity, 1*(2), 117. https://doi.org/10.1037/sgd0000032

Fattoracci, E. S. M., Revels-Macalinao, M., & Huynh, Q. L. (2020). Greater than the sum of racism and heterosexism: Intersectional microaggressions toward racial/ethnic and sexual minority group members. *Cultural Diversity and Ethnic Minority Psychology*. Published online ahead of print. https://doi.org/10.1037/cdp0000329.

Flanders, C. E., Shuler, S. A., Desnoyers, S. A., & VanKim, N. A. (2019). Relationships between social support, identity, anxiety, and depression among young bisexual people of color. *Journal of Bisexuality*. https://doi.org/10.108 0/15299716.2019.1617543

Ghabrial, M. A. (2017). "Trying to figure out where we belong:" narratives of racialized sexual minorities on community, identity, discrimination, and health.

Sexuality Research and Social Policy, 14(1), 42–55. https://doi.org/10.1007/s13178-016-0229-x

Gray, N. N., Mendelsohn, D. M., & Omoto, A. M. (2015). Community connectedness, conflict, stress, and resilience among gay Latino immigrants. *American Journal of Community Psychology, 55*(1–2), 202–214. https://doi.org/10.1007/s10464-014-9697-4

Harris, A., Battle, J., Pastrana, A., & Daniels, J. (2015). Feelings of belonging: An exploratory analysis of the sociopolitical involvement of Black, Latina, and Asian/Pacific islander sexual minority women. *Journal of Homosexuality, 62*(10), 1374–1397. https://doi.org/10.1080/00918369.2015.1061360

Hatzenbuehler, M. L. (2009). How does sexual minority stigma "get under the skin?": A psychological mediation framework. *Psychological Bulletin, 135*(5), 707. https://doi.org/10.1037/a0016441

Kattari, S. K., Walls, N. E., Whitfield, D. L., & Magruder, L. L. (2017). Racial and ethnic differences in experiences of discrimination in accessing social services among transgender/gender-nonconforming people. *Journal of Ethnic & Cultural Diversity in Social Work: Innovation in Theory, Research & Practice, 26*(3), 217–235. https://doi.org/10.1080/15313204.2016.1242102

Li, M. J., Thing, J. P., Galvan, F. H., Gonzalez, K. D., & Bluthenthal, R. N. (2017). Contextualising family microaggressions and strategies of resilience among young gay and bisexual men of Latino heritage. *Culture. Health & Sexuality, 19*(1), 107–120. https://doi.org/10.1080/13691058.2016.1208273

Lira, A. N., & Morais, N. A. (2017). Resilience in lesbian, gay, and bisexual (LGB) populations: An integrative literature review. *Sexuality Research & Social Policy: A Journal of the NSRC.* https://doi.org/10.1007/s13178-017-0285-x

Mayer, K. H., Wang, L., Koblin, B., Mannheimer, S., Magnus, M., Del Rio, C., ... Piwowar-Manning, E. (2014). Concomitant socioeconomic, behavioral, and biological factors associated with the disproportionate HIV infection burden among Black men who have sex with men in 6 US cities. *PLoS One, 9*(1), 1–10. https://doi.org/10.1371/journal.pone.0087298

Meyer, I. H. (2003). Prejudice, social stress, and mental health in lesbian, gay, and bisexual populations: Conceptual issues and research evidence. *Psychological Bulletin, 129*, 674–697. https://doi.org/10.1037/0033-2909.129.5.674

Moradi, B., DeBlaere, C., & Huang, Y. P. (2010). Centralizing the experiences of LGB people of color in counseling psychology 1Ψ7. *The Counseling Psychologist, 38*(3), 322–330. https://doi.org/10.1177/0011000008330832

Moradi, B., Wiseman, M. C., DeBlaere, C., Goodman, M. B., Sarkees, A., Brewster, M. E., & Huang, Y. P. (2010). LGB of color and white individuals' perceptions of heterosexist stigma, internalized homophobia, and outness: Comparisons of levels and links. *The Counseling Psychologist, 38*(3), 397–424. https://doi.org/10.1177/0011000009335263

Mosley, D., Abreu, R. L., & Crowell, C. (2017). Resistance as resilience: How the Black bisexual community keeps one another healthy. In L. D. Follins & J. M. Lassiter (Eds.), *Black LGBT health in the United States: The intersection of race, gender, and sexual orientation* (pp. 55–72). Lanham, MD: The Rowman & Littefield Publishing Group.

NIH. (2020). National institute on minority health and health disparities: Overview. Retrieved from https://www.nimhd.nih.gov/about/overview/

Ouch, S., & Moradi, B. (2019). Cognitive and affective expectation of stigma, coping efficacy, and psychological distress among sexual minority people of color. *Journal of Counseling Psychology, 66*(4), 424–436. https://doi.org/10.1037/cou0000360

Perrin, P. B., Sutter, M. E., Trujillo, M. A., Henry, R. S., & Pugh, M., Jr. (2020). The minority strengths model: Development and initial path analytic validation in racially/ethnically diverse LGBTQ individuals. *Journal of Clinical Psychology, 76*(1), 118–136. https://doi.org/10.1002/jclp.22850

Purdie-Vaughns, V., & Eibach, R. P. (2008). Intersectional invisibility: The distinctive advantages and disadvantages of multiple subordinate-group identities. *Sex Roles, 59*(5–6), 377–391. https://doi.org/10.1007/s11199-008-9424-4

Ryan, C., Huebner, D., Diaz, R. M., & Sanchez, J. (2009). Family rejection as a predictor of negative health outcomes in white and Latino lesbian, gay, and bisexual young adults. *Pediatrics, 123*, 346–352. https://doi.org/10.1542/peds.2007-3524

Sadika, B., Wiebe, E., Morrison, M. A., & Morrison, T. G. (2020). Intersectional microaggressions and social support for LGBTQ persons of color: A systematic review of the Canadian-based empirical literature. *Journal of GLBT Family Studies.* https://doi.org/10.1080/1550428X.2020.1724125

Scandurra, C., Amodeo, A. L., Valerio, P., Bochicchio, V., & Frost, D. M. (2017). Minority stress, resilience, and mental health: A study of Italian transgender people. *Journal of Social Issues, 73*(3), 563–585. https://doi.org/10.1111/josi.12232

Schwartz, D. R., Stratton, N., & Hart, T. A. (2016). Minority stress and mental and sexual health: Examining the psychological mediation framework among gay and bisexual men. *Psychology of Sexual Orientation and Gender Diversity, 3*(3), 313–324. https://doi.org/10.1037/sgd0000180

Shin, R. Q., Welch, J. C., Kaya, A. E., Yeung, J. G., Obana, C., Sharma, R., … Yee, S. (2017). The intersectionality framework and identity intersections in the journal of counseling psychology and the counseling psychologist: A content analysis. *Journal of Counseling Psychology, 64*(5), 458–474. https://doi.org/10.1037/cou0000204

Singh, A. A. (2013). Transgender youth of color and resilience: Negotiating oppression and finding support. *Sex Roles, 68*(11–12), 690–702. https://doi.org/10.1007/s11199-012-0149-z

Singh, A. A., & McKleroy, V. S. (2011). "Just getting out of bed is a revolutionary act": The resilience of transgender people of color who have survived traumatic life events. *Traumatology, 17*(2), 34–44. https://doi.org/10.1177/1534765610369261

Stone, A. L., Nimmons, E. A., Salcido, R., & Schnarrs, P. (2020). "My meemaw is a cool ass person:" family members as role models of resilience for sexual and gender diverse people of color. *Journal of GLBT Family Studies.* https://doi.org/10.1080/1550428X.2020.1724148

Substance Abuse and Mental Health Service Administration. (2020). 2018 National Survey on Drug Use and health: Lesbian, gay, & bisexual (LGB) Adults. Retrieved from https://www.samhsa.gov/data/report/2018-nsduh-lesbian-gay-bisexual-lgb-adults

Sutter, M., & Perrin, P. B. (2016). Discrimination, mental health, and suicidal ideation among LGBTQ people of color. *Journal of Counseling Psychology, 63*(1), 98–105. https://doi.org/10.1037/cou0000126

Szymanski, D. M., & Gupta, A. (2009). Examining the relationship between multiple internalized oppressions and African American lesbian, gay, bisexual, and questioning persons' self-esteem and psychological distress. *Journal of Counseling Psychology, 56*(1), 110–118. https://doi.org/10.1037/a0012981

The Trevor Project. (2020). *2020 National Survey on LGBTQ Youth Mental Health.* Retrieved from https://www.thetrevorproject.org/survey-2020/

Vaughan, M. D., Miles, J., Parent, M. C., Lee, H. S., Tilghman, J. D., & Prokhorets, S. (2014). A content analysis of LGBT-themed positive psychology articles. *Psychology of Sexual Orientation and Gender Diversity, 1*(4), 313–324. https://doi.org/10.1037/sgd0000060

Velez, B. L., Polihronakis, C. J., Watson, L. B., & Cox, R., Jr. (2019). Heterosexism, racism, and the mental health of sexual minority people of color. *The Counseling Psychologist, 47*(1), 129–159. https://doi.org/10.1177/0011000019828309

Wong, F. Y. (2015). In search for the many faces of community resilience among LGBT individuals. *American Journal of Community Psychology, 55*(1–2), 239–241. https://doi.org/10.1007/s10464-015-9703-5

PART V

Conclusions

CHAPTER 11

Resilience in LGBTQ PoC

Benjamin Aguilera and Aldo Barrita

Abstract LGBTQ People of Color (PoC) experience chronic oppression and their ability to survive these experiences is often attributed to their remarkable resilience. This chapter analyzes theoretical models focused on resilience for sexual/gender minority PoC. In particular, how LGBTQ PoC experience individual and community resilience is explored. Moreover, frameworks such as syndemics are discussed, and themes related to intersectionality and religiosity are highlighted as a societal-level factor pertaining to resilience building for LGBTQ PoC. Together, this chapter serves as a summary of findings on resilience in LGBTQ PoC, while also providing a critique and suggestions for future research in the study of resilience with racial/ethnic LGBTQ communities.

B. Aguilera (✉)
Department of Psychology, University of La Verne, La Verne, CA, USA
e-mail: benjamin.aguilera@laverne.edu

A. Barrita
Department of Psychology, University of Nevada, Las Vegas,
Las Vegas, NV, USA
e-mail: barrita@unlv.nevada.edu

Keywords Resilience • Individual and community • Intersectionality • Religiosity

Lesbian, Gay, Bisexual, Transgender, and Queer (LGBTQ) People of Color (PoC) experience chronic oppression (Nadal, 2019) and their ability to survive these experiences is often attributed to their remarkable resilience. However, a specific examination of resilience within LGBTQ PoC is missing in research. Perhaps the reason for this is that there are complexities inherent with navigating society as a person with multiple marginalized identities (i.e., as a racial/ethnic and sexual/gender-diverse person). In particular, societal stigma and marginalization create adverse social environments that make it difficult for racial/ethnic sexual/gender minorities to exist as social beings (Nadal, 2019). Relatedly, the intersectional experiences of these identities for LGBTQ PoC requires an examination of how resilience is defined, with whom resilience research has been conducted with, and what expectations researchers have with the concept of resilience for racial/ethnic LGBTQ.

This chapter will explore theoretical models focused on resilience for sexual/gender minority (SGM) PoC. In particular, how LGBTQ PoC experience individual and community resilience will be explored. Moreover, frameworks such as syndemics will be discussed, and themes related to intersectionality and religiosity will be highlighted as societal-level factor as they relate to resilience building for LGBTQ PoC. This chapter serves as a summary of findings on resilience in LGBTQ PoC, as well as providing a critique and suggestions for future research in the study of resilience with racial/ethnic SGM communities.

DEFINING RESILIENCE: LITERATURE AND FRAMEWORKS

Resilience is often conceptualized as a buffer that lessens the impact of stress in the face of adversity (McConnell, Janulis, Phillips II, Truong, & Birkett, 2018). However, multiple definitions of resilience exist, all of which attempt to capture how resilience works in LGBTQ PoC communities. For example, Wilson et al. (2016) conceptualize resilience as models of *protective, compensatory,* and *challenge.* The protective model of resilience states that the individual utilizes psychological resources to minimize or eliminate a threat. Indeed, McConnell et al. (2018) view resilience as a protective model against stressors individuals face, reducing the stress response in the face of a threat. In contrast, the compensatory model describes resilience as physical, emotional, and psychological actions done to overcome adversity regardless of how high such adversity is. Lastly, the challenge framework posits that level of adversity is related to whether or not there are positive outcomes; if a person faces high levels of adversity, overcoming hardships with resilience may not be possible (Wilson et al., 2016). These models individually attempt to define resilience; however, Freitas, Coimbra, and Fontaine (2017), in a systematic review across 13 studies, found that there is supporting evidence for each conceptualization of resilience. Thus, defining resilience depends on which model is used to accurately represent the multidimensional experiences of resilience for racial/ethnic LGBTQ (Freitas et al., 2017; Woodward, Banks, Marks, & Pantalone, 2017).

While positive psychology research shows that positive emotions can improve a person's resilience (Domínguez, Bobele, Coppock, & Peña, 2015), little research has examined how resilience helps LGBTQ communities overcome or handle adversity. A recent integrative review (De Lira & Morais, 2018) documents what resilience looks like for sexual minorities (i.e., LGB) across 39 studies. In particular, they found that resilience sources for sexual minorities fall into three sources: individual, family, and community-based. Furthermore, main risk factors against developing resilience include homophobia and concealment of sexual orientation, whereas protective factors included emotional openness, family support, and spirituality.

To this end, there is a need for a theoretical framework that captures resilience for sexual minority PoC. Perhaps the positive psychology framework may be useful, given its focus on community relatedness. For example, the LGBTQ relationally-based positive psychology framework (Domínguez et al., 2015) is an example of such a framework that uses a strengths-based perspective, systematic orientation of family resilience, and draws from LGBTQ family literature regarding resilience and community relatedness. Importantly, this framework highlights that heteronormativity impacts how resilience is viewed in non-heterosexual families and couples. Although the positive psychology LGBTQ framework examines resilience for LGBTQ individuals, limitations include no examination of those typically less represented such as Trans and Gender-Non-Conforming persons (TGNC) racial/ethnic persons (Testa, Habarth, Peta, Balsam, & Bockting, 2015). Thus, frameworks that center the experiences of both racial/ethnic and sexual/gender minority identities are much needed.

INDIVIDUAL AND COMMUNITY RESILIENCE

Many factors contribute to the health and well-being of racial/ethnic SGMs, including trauma, internalized homophobia, and coping with everyday stressors (Meyer, 2010). These factors also contribute to both individual and community-level resilience. In terms of defining resilience for LGBTQ PoC, it is important to make a distinction between individual and community-level resilience. Individual resilience is defined as how a person is able to achieve or sustain health and well-being in the face of adversity or avoiding the risk altogether, by taking risk-protective factors into account (Shilo, Antebi, & Mor, 2015). Assessment tools for TGNC communities, namely the Gender Minority Stress and Resilience (GMSR) measure, have been created to explore individual-level resilience for these communities (Testa et al., 2015). In contrast, community-level resilience is operationalized as the resources or attributes that operate as external forces that impact individuals at a community level (Shilo et al., 2015). Community resilience for LGBTQ individuals includes social support and community connectedness from the LGBTQ community (De Lira & Morais, 2018), which provide positive social support and experiences for LGBTQ persons. Support systems, especially at the community level such as LGBQ connectedness with friends and partners or family support, are important to promote well-being and serve as buffers against mental distress in both LGBQ youth and adults (Shilo et al., 2015). Although there is extensive evidence on resilience, both individual and community resilience research does not center the intersectional experiences of LGBTQ who have other marginalized identities (e.g., differing socioeconomic statuses, those who live in substandard housing, race, gender), which makes it difficult to know how people with multiple minoritized statuses use and access sources of resilience at both levels.

A framework that highlights how LGBTQ PoC may experience community-level resilience differently than white LGBTQ is syndemics, which refers to overlapping epidemic or community-level factors that affect an individual (Latkin, German, Vlahov, & Galea, 2013) such as poverty, discrimination, and racism, and other experiences salient to socially minoritized identities. To illustrate this, Wilson et al. (2016) used the framework of syndemics to understand resilience in young Black gay and bisexual men and found different profiles of resilience among these groups, given they are disproportionately affected by increased HIV/AIDS risk and poverty. The framework of syndemics suggests that the combination of these factors act collectively to create higher-risk environments for those with already marginalized identities (e.g., trans women of color), which result in substandard living conditions that impact their health and quality of life. More importantly, the syndemics framework proposes that resilience is not a "one size fits all" phenomenon, especially when examining individuals with various marginalized identities such as LGBTQ PoC. For example, Black and Native Americans TGNC individuals report connecting with LGBTQ PoC communities but do not find the same connection with the broader white LGBTQ community (Stone, Nimmons, Salcido, & Schnarrs, 2020). As a result, perhaps the syndemics framework provides a nuanced examination of this integral factor for LGBTQ PoC. That is, if the collective totality of risk factors experienced by LGBTQ PoC is not considered, then the resilience frameworks currently available will not accurately capture or represent the true lived experiences of racial/ethnic LGBTQ. Thus, it is necessary to include the syndemics framework when assessing resilience for LGBTQ PoC.

INTERSECTIONALITY AND RESILIENCE

LGBTQ PoC exist at the intersection of their social identities (e.g., race, gender, sexual identity, education, SES). As a result, it is important to acknowledge the influence of multiple sources of social marginalization of their identities that make unique lived intersectional experiences for these groups. Intersectionality theory posits that different aspects of an individual's life intersect and interact with each other, especially with marginalized identities (Crenshaw, 2017). To illustrate the importance of this, McConnell et al. (2018) used both minority stress theory and intersectionality theory to examine stress-related experiences for Black gay and bisexual men and found that a nuanced perspective related to living at the intersections of more than one marginalized identity exposes people to intersectional discrimination as a source of stress. To further illustrate the unique impact of intersectional discrimination, Fattoracci, Revels-Macalinao, and Huynh (2020) developed a scale that measures both racial and sexual minority microaggressions for LGBTQ PoC. Their findings show that solely utilizing minority stress theory to conceptualize resilience in LGBTQ PoC does not capture the combined and unique lived social realities of racism and heterosexism. Thus, intersectionality provides a unique perspective on social identities and coinciding experiences of LGBTQ PoC that fully captures their unique resilience.

Exploring resilience from an intersectional lens has allowed literature to move past individual resilience frameworks and develop theories of community resilience that highlight the importance of community context of TGNC PoC well-being (Singh, 2017; Stone et al., 2020). Intersectional approaches also show that groups like gay Latino immigrants experience specific immigration-related stressors and support that influence their resilience-building from community sources (Gray, Mendelsohn, & Omoto, 2015). Moreover, bisexual PoC who have less social support experience greater binegativity, anxiety, and depressive symptoms (Flanders, Shuler, Desnoyers, & VanKim, 2019). Thus, intersectionality provides an intricate framework that best captures resilience, as it considers societal marginalization in the form of intersectional discrimination for LGBTQ PoC.

A focus on intersectionality in the study of resilience can be even more important for specific groups within LGBTQ PoC (Follins, Walker, & Lewis, 2014), such as Transgender Women of Color (TWoC). Singh and McKleroy (2011) found that TWoC who have survived traumatic life events also experienced high levels of transphobia and racism. Yet, they also reported feeling pride in TWoC identity, which is crucial to developing resilience. These findings support the Transgender Resilience Intervention Model (TRIM; Matsuno & Israel, 2018), which indicates self-acceptance and pride as positive predictors of individual-level resilience. The TRIM also addresses other factors for resilience such as positive role models, community, and family support. More specifically, Singh and McKleroy (2011) found family support was an important part of community resilience when transgender PoC feel acceptance for both of their identities (race and gender). Intersectional frameworks show that for TWoC resilience, adverse conditions and coping resources are important (White, 2013). Perhaps this is most salient in recent dissertations by young scholars in the field. For example, African-American transgender women who reported high levels of violent experiences (systemic, physical, and verbal) counter these experiences by drawing from both individual and community-level resilience and coping strategies (LaMartine, 2020). Similarly, TGNC Latinx immigrants seeking asylum who are detained in the U.S. who experience abuse and transphobia remarkably harness individual and community-level resilience in the form of solidarity and support from other detainees (Minero, 2020). Thus, recent work centering intersectionality with LGBTQ PoC sheds light on the diverse forms of resilience demonstrated by these communities in different contexts.

Religiosity/Spirituality as Resilience

Despite the complicated relationship between LGBTQ PoC and religion (Coley, 2017), racial/ethnic LGBTQ groups often utilize their spirituality and religion as a source of individual and community-level resilience (De Lira & Morais, 2018). Yet, LGBTQ who seek support from a religious institution that does not support their identities experience greater mental health issues (Coley, 2017). Moreover, older LGB adults who grew up in heterosexist faith environments feel inferior and internalize LGB oppression (Bourn, Frantell, & Miles, 2018), particularly gay and bisexual men developing internalized shame and guilt (Lassiter et al., 2017). Although spirituality and religion overlap, spirituality is often described as the ongoing search for the sacred *divine* aspect of life, while religion is described as the search for significance that occurs in institutions that facilitate spirituality (Lassiter et al., 2019). Majority of the research on religion and spirituality as a form of resilience for LGBTQ has used racially mixed samples, and only a few studies have highlighted differences for LGBTQ PoC. Specifically, TWoC use spiritual resilience to counter psychological effects from traumatic life events (Singh & McKleroy, 2011). Additionally, Walker and Longmire-Avital (2013) found that young Black LGB use their religion as a tool to cope, often indicating that religion provides a sense of hope and perseverance. These findings suggest further research on religious/spiritual practices and engagement, as a form of resilience, especially focused on LGBTQ PoC.

A Critique on Resilience and Related Research

As demonstrated, the field is moving toward examining resilience in LGBTQ populations, with some studies specifically focused on LGBTQ PoC. However, it is apparent that critiquing how researchers conceptualize, measure, and operationalize resilience from their theoretical frameworks in literature is needed. To successfully harness LGBTQ PoC resilience to promote heart, brain, and mental health, the field must examine these questions to accurately capture the resilience experience of LGBTQ PoC. Moreover, the gaps in current literature make it challenging to successfully measure resilience and explore what it means to be resilient as a racial/ethnic LGBTQ person.

Although resilience is posited to be an important factor in the lives of LGBTQ PoC, this construct is still largely under-researched (Wilson et al.,

2016). The limitations of resilience frameworks are important when considering the complexities that accompany research involving LGBTQ PoC. Intersectionality theory and minority stress theory (Crenshaw, 2017; McConnell et al., 2018) suggest the consideration of the collective toll of multiple marginalized identities or the influence of systematic oppression from dominant groups when assessing mechanisms of resilience for LGBTQ PoC; however, this is missing from the literature. Another limitation in resilience research pertaining to LGBTQ PoC is the lack of longitudinal studies to examine factors like intersectional stigma and resilience across time, which may shed light on how patterns of intersectional stress are associated with resilience. This longitudinal approach has been preliminarily examined in recent research with Black LGBQ people, where negative experiences of intersectional discrimination were associated with negative affect (as mediated by identity conflict and rumination) over the span of a week using a daily diary method (Jackson, Mohr, Sarno, Kindahl, & Jones, 2020); however, resilience as a variable was not directly tested.

A lack of theory-driven frameworks used, coupled with limited ways to measure LGBTQ PoC resilience, is salient in the research. Indeed, most studies employ qualitative methods as a way of measurement of resilience in PoC because of limited validated scales and measures in the field (Salahuddin & O'Brien, 2011). This leaves researchers to conceptualize the unique experiences of LGBTQ PoC within the confines of broader LGBTQ resilience frameworks. Lacking focus on issues like intersectional stress prevents the discovery of variables that could lead to positive resilience in specific communities like transgender PoC (Breslow et al., 2015). This does a disservice to people who hold multiple socially minoritized identities, by placing limits on the totality of their experiences.

In a broader sense, it is important to discuss what it means to study resilience as coping in the context of intersectional discrimination. In particular, does the literature suggest that resilience is an approach that LGBTQ PoC should use to cope with experiences of intersectional discrimination? If said resilience frameworks suggest that LGBTQ PoC need to develop resilience in the face of racism and discrimination, such a suggestion does not directly tackle systems of oppression and marginalization; rather, this approach places the responsibility of adapting to institutional and systemic racism and heterosexism on LGBT PoC. Although viewing resilience in this way is well intentioned and has practical clinical implications, it is also harmful and problematic, as it misses the opportunity to tackle the true root causes of racism, heterosexism, transphobia, biphobia, and homophobia experienced by LGBT PoC in societies.

FUTURE DIRECTIONS

Resilience in LGBTQ PoC is a complex phenomenon that requires greater investigation to accurately represent intersectional experiences. The limited availability of measures, intentional recruitment of LGBTQ PoC in resilience research, and theoretical frameworks specifically designed for LGBTQ PoC impede a strong understanding of resilience for these communities. Though much remains unexplored, some work and theories have contributed to the limited understanding of LGBTQ PoC resilience. Intersectionality theory, minority stress theory, and syndemics are frameworks integral to conceptualizing resilience experienced by LGBTQ PoC. Before harnessing resilience in LGBTQ PoC to promote heart, brain, and mental health, other resilience frameworks salient to LGBTQ PoC must be explored, in order to accurately portray their resilience experience in the scientific literature. This is important, as LGBTQ PoC experience marginalization from society and this is perpetuated by what gets published in the sciences. Therefore, it is incumbent on researchers to provide justice to these communities by accurately assessing and describing their lived experiences and sources of resilience.

REFERENCES

Bourn, J. R., Frantell, K. A., & Miles, J. R. (2018). Internalized heterosexism, religious coping, and psychache in LGB young adults who identify as religious. *Psychology of Sexual Orientation and Gender Diversity, 5*(3), 303–312. https://doi.org/10.1037/sgd0000274

Breslow, A. S., Brewster, M. E., Velez, B. L., Wong, S., Geiger, E., & Soderstrom, B. (2015). Resilience and collective action: Exploring buffers against minority stress for transgender individuals. *Psychology of Sexual Orientation and Gender Diversity, 2*(3), 253–265. https://doi.org/10.1037/sgd0000117

Coley, J. S. (2017). Reconciling religion and LGBT rights: Christian universities, theological orientations, and LGBT inclusion. *Social Currents, 4*(1), 87–106. https://doi.org/10.1177/2329496516651639

Crenshaw, K. W. (2017). *On intersectionality: Essential writings*. The New Press.

De Lira, A. N., & Morais, N. A. (2018). Resilience in lesbian, gay, and bisexual (LGB) populations: An integrative literature review. *Sexuality Research and Social Policy, 15*(3), 272–282. https://doi.org/10.1007/s13178-017-0285-x

146   B. AGUILERA AND A. BARRITA

Domínguez, D. G., Bobele, M., Coppock, J., & Peña, E. (2015). LGBTQ relationally based positive psychology: An inclusive and systemic framework. *Psychological Services, 12*(2), 177–185. https://doi.org/10.1037/a0038824

Fattoracci, E. S. M., Revels-Macalinao, M., & Huynh, Q.L. (2020). Greater than the sum of racism and heterosexism: Intersectional microaggressions toward racial/ethnic and sexual minority group members. *Cultural Diversity and Ethnic Minority Psychology*. Published online ahead of print. https://doi.org/10.1037/cdp0000329.

Flanders, C. E., Shuler, S. A., Desnoyers, S. A., & VanKim, N. A. (2019). Relationships between social support, identity, anxiety, and depression among young bisexual people of color. *Journal of Bisexuality, 19*(2), 253–275. https://doi.org/10.1080/15299716.2019.1617543

Follins, L. D., Walker, J. J., & Lewis, M. K. (2014). Resilience in black lesbian, gay, bisexual, and transgender individuals: A critical review of the literature. *Journal of Gay & Lesbian Mental Health, 18*(2), 190–212. https://doi.org/10.1080/19359705.2013.828343

Freitas, D. F., Coimbra, S., & Fontaine, A. M. (2017). Resilience in LGB youths: A systematic review of protection mechanisms. *Paidéia (Ribeirão Preto), 27*(66), 69–79. https://doi.org/10.1590/1982-43272766201709

Gray, N. N., Mendelsohn, D. M., & Omoto, A. M. (2015). Community connectedness, challenges, and resilience among gay Latino immigrants. *American Journal of Community Psychology, 55*(1–2), 202–214. https://doi.org/10.1007/s10464-014-9697-4

Jackson, S. D., Mohr, J. J., Sarno, E. L., Kindahl, A. M., & Jones, I. L. (2020). Intersectional experiences, stigma-related stress, and psychological health among black LGBQ individuals. *Journal of Consulting and Clinical Psychology, 88*(5), 416–428. https://doi.org/10.1037/ccp0000489

LaMartine, S. (2020). *Experiences of violence, victimization, and coping among African American transgender women*. Retrieved from ProQuest Dissertations & Theses Global. (28022144).

Lassiter, J. M., Saleh, L., Grov, C., Starks, T., Ventuneac, A., & Parsons, J. T. (2019). Spirituality and multiple dimensions of religion are associated with mental health in gay and bisexual men: Results from the one thousand strong cohort. *Psychology of Religion and Spirituality, 11*(4), 408–416. https://doi.org/10.1037/rel0000146

Lassiter, J. M., Saleh, L., Starks, T., Grov, C., Ventuneac, A., & Parsons, J. T. (2017). Race, ethnicity, religious affiliation, and education are associated with gay and bisexual men's religious and spiritual participation and beliefs: Results from the one thousand strong cohort. *Cultural Diversity and Ethnic Minority Psychology, 23*(4), 468–476. https://doi.org/10.1037/cdp0000143

Latkin, C. A., German, D., Vlahov, D., & Galea, S. (2013). Neighborhoods and HIV: A social ecological approach to prevention and care. *American Psychologist, 68*(4), 210–224. https://doi.org/10.1037/a0032704

Matsuno, E., & Israel, T. (2018). Psychological interventions promoting resilience among transgender individuals: Transgender resilience intervention model (TRIM). *The Counseling Psychologist, 46*(5), 632–655. https://doi. org/10.1177/0011000018787261

McConnell, E. A., Janulis, P., Phillips, G., II, Truong, R., & Birkett, M. (2018). Multiple minority stress and LGBT community resilience among sexual minority men. *Psychology of Sexual Orientation and Gender Diversity, 5*(1), 1–12. https://doi.org/10.1037/sgd0000265

Meyer, I. H. (2010). Identity, stress, and resilience in lesbians, gay men, and bisexuals of color. *The Counseling Psychologist, 38*(3), 442–454. https://doi. org/10.1177/0011000009351601

Minero, L. P. (2020). *The impact of detention proceedings and solitary confinement on Latinx, transgender, undocumented and asylum seeking immigrants.* Retrieved from ProQuest Dissertations & Theses Global. (29028900).

Nadal, K. L. (2019). A decade of microaggression research and LGBTQ communities: An introduction to the special issue. *Journal of Homosexuality, 66*(10), 1309–1316. https://doi.org/10.1080/00918369.2018.1539582

Salahuddin, N. M., & O'Brien, K. M. (2011). Challenges and resilience in the lives of urban, multiracial adults: An instrument development study. *Journal of Counseling Psychology, 58*(4), 494–507. https://doi.org/10.1037/a0024633

Shilo, G., Antebi, N., & Mor, Z. (2015). Individual and community resilience factors among lesbian, gay, bisexual, queer and questioning youth and adults in Israel. *American Journal of Community Psychology, 55*(1–2), 215–227. https:// doi.org/10.1007/s10464-014-9693-8

Singh A. A. (2017). Understanding trauma and supporting resilience with LGBT people of color. In K. Eckstrand & J. Potter (Eds.), *Trauma, Resilience, and health promotion in LGBT patients.* Springer. https://doi. org/10.1007/978-3-319-54509-7_10.

Singh, A. A., & McKleroy, V. S. (2011). "Just getting out of bed is a revolutionary act:" the resilience of transgender people of color who have survived traumatic life events. *Traumatology, 17*(2), 34–44. https://doi.org/10.1177/1534765610369261

Stone, A. L., Nimmons, E. A., Salcido, R., Jr., & Schnarrs, P. W. (2020). Multiplicity, race, and resilience: Transgender and non-binary people building community. *Sociological Inquiry, 90*(2), 226–248.

Testa, R. J., Habarth, J., Peta, J., Balsam, K., & Bockting, W. (2015). Development of the gender minority stress and resilience measure. *Psychology of Sexual Orientation and Gender Diversity, 2*(1), 65–77. https://doi.org/10.1037/sgd0000081

Walker, J. J., & Longmire-Avital, B. (2013). The impact of religious faith and internalized homonegativity on resiliency for black lesbian, gay, and bisexual emerging adults. *Developmental Psychology, 49*(9), 1723–1731. https://doi. org/10.1037/a0031059

White, M. G. (2013). *Resiliency factors among transgender people of color.* Retrieved from UWM Digital Commons Theses and Dissertations. Retrieved from https://dc.uwm.edu/etf/182

Wilson, P. A., Meyer, I. H., Antebi-Gruszka, N., Boone, M. R., Cook, S. H., & Cherenack, E. M. (2016). Profiles of resilience and psychosocial outcomes among young black gay and bisexual men. *American Journal of Community Psychology, 57*(1–2), 144–157. https://doi.org/10.1002/ajcp.12018

Woodward, E. N., Banks, R. J., Marks, A. K., & Pantalone, D. W. (2017). Identifying resilience resources for HIV prevention among sexual minority men: A systematic review. *AIDS and Behavior, 21*(10), 2860–2873. https://doi.org/10.1007/s10461-016-1608-2

CHAPTER 12

Structural Stigma and LGBTQ PoC Health

Amy Prescott, Matthew Alcala, and Nadine Nakamura

Abstract Throughout history, the United States has enacted numerous federal and state policies that have greatly impacted the health and well-being of LGBTQ individuals by perpetuating structural stigma. This chapter starts by highlighting the inequities of structural stigma for LGBTQ people, arguing that there are limited data available about LGBTQ PoC. Next, the insidious impact of structural stigma on health is explored in this study, with findings highlighted for LGBTQ PoC, across a variety of diseases and social contexts. The chapter ends with key future directions, particularly state initiatives, that can positively impact LGBTQ PoC health.

Keywords Structural Stigma • LGBTQ PoC health disparities • Health Equity

A. Prescott (✉) • M. Alcala • N. Nakamura
Department of Psychology, University of La Verne, La Verne, CA, USA
e-mail: amy.prescott@laverne.edu; matthew.alcala@laverne.edu; nnakamura@laverne.edu

© The Author(s), under exclusive license to Springer Nature
Switzerland AG 2021
J. J. García (ed.), *Heart, Brain and Mental Health Disparities for LGBTQ People of Color*,
https://doi.org/10.1007/978-3-030-70060-7_12

149

Throughout history, the United States has enacted numerous federal and state policies that have greatly impacted the health and well-being of Lesbian, Gay, Bisexual, Transgender, and Queer (LGBTQ) individuals by perpetuating *structural stigma*. Structural stigma refers to the policies of private and governmental institutions that hinder stigmatized individuals by limiting access to opportunities and resources, as well as societal expectations that further enforce these oppressive policies (Hatzenbuehler, 2014). However, the devastating impact of structural stigma on LGBTQ PoC specifically will be centered and explored in this chapter.

POLICIES IMPACTING LGBTQ PEOPLE

To understand why structural stigma disproportionately impacts LGBTQ PoC, there must first be an overview on the impacts of this type of stigma on the broader LGBTQ community. Indeed, structural stigma against LGBTQ people has existed in a variety of forms, including anti-sodomy laws, immigration exclusions, and government employment discrimination (Hatzenbuehler, 2014). However, LGBTQ people have fought back against discriminatory policies through advocacy, legislative efforts, and legal challenges. The first major federal legislation proposed to uphold LGBTQ rights was the 1974 Equality Act, which would have amended the Civil Rights Act of 1964 to include prohibition of discrimination on the basis of sex assigned at birth, sexual orientation, and marital status in federally assisted programs, housing and financial services (Human Rights Campaign [HRC], 2020b). Additional advancements in LGBTQ rights have been made, particularly in the areas of marriage equality and anti-discrimination policies (HRC, 2020a). Moreover, the nation's largest safety net health-care system, the Veteran Health Administration, has created specific directives with policies and procedures to provide LGBTQ affirmative health care (U.S. Department of Veteran Affairs, 2020). Nonetheless, as efforts to be inclusive are made, new discriminatory policies are also put forth, including former President Trump's ban on transgender individuals in the military, withdrawal of protection for transgender students under Title IX, and halting enforcement of the Affordable Care Act's nondiscrimination protections for transgender people (National Center for Transgender Equality, 2020).

Structural Stigma and LGBTQ Health Disparities

In general, LGBTQ rights impact the health and well-being of these communities. For example, Wight and colleagues (2013) found no mental health disparities between LGB and heterosexuals in states that recognized same-sex marriage prior to the Supreme Court decision, indicating that having basic rights to marry as LGBTQ persons may have promoted the mental health of these communities. Moreover, the largest improvement in psychological health (from negative to positive outcomes) for LGBTQ adult was found among those residents in states where same-sex marriages were not recognized prior to the Supreme Court decision (Flores, Mallory, & Conron, 2020). Comparatively, negative psychological symptoms are significantly higher among LGB individuals living in states with policies that do not protect sexual/gender minorities (SGMs) from hate crimes and employment discrimination (Hatzenbuehler, 2014). To corroborate this assertion, researchers found that the more stigmatizing policies a state has (e.g. banning same-sex marriage), the higher the risk for smoking and drinking among gay and bisexual men and an increased illicit drug use in LGB youth (Hatzenbuehler, Jun, Corliss, & Bryn Austin, 2015; Pachankis, Hatzenbuehler, & Starks, 2014).

Similar trends for the impact of structural stigma on health are seen among transgender populations; however, there is limited literature. For example, in their analysis of state-level policies, Perez-Brumer, Hatzenbuehler, Oldenburg, and Bockting (2015) found that a reduction in structural stigma was associated with reduced odds of suicide and suicide attempts in a sample of transwomen and transmen. Given similarities in outcomes for stigma, it is probable that transgender populations also experience poorer health due to structural stigma (Hughto, Reisner, & Pachankis, 2015). However, these effects have been understudied by race/ethnicity within transgender samples. A recent study by Goldenberg, Reisner, Harper, Gamarel, and Stephenson (2020) found more instances of healthcare avoidance due to fear of mistreatment within specific groups of transgender people of color (PoC; 36% of American Indian/Alaskan Native participants, 23% of Asian, Native Hawaiian, Pacific Islander participants, 25% of Black participants, and 25% of Latinx/Hispanic participants), compared to white participants. These findings provide data on the impact of structural stigma and health for gender minorities, including the important role of protective federal policies and improved health for these communities. They also indicate greater experiences of structural stigma adversely impact health. However, much of the research on structural stigma focuses on white LGB, with few studies centering on race/ethnicity. Thus, it is imperative for research on structural stigma to make comparisons not only by sexual orientation/gender identity, but also by race and ethnicity.

STRUCTURAL STIGMA AND LGBTQ PoC HEALTH DISPARITIES

To this end, it is important to center racial/ethnic LGBTQ. These communities not only experience the devastating impact of anti-LGBTQ laws and policies, but also face the insidious and chronic impacts of racism (Fredriksen-Goldsen et al., 2013). Research on the role of structural racism in terms of health of LGBTQ PoC, as well as the impact of minority stress on the brain health of LGBT elders, suggests these sources of stigma have cumulative and intersectional impacts on LGBTQ PoC heart and brain health (Correro II & Nielson, 2020; Lukachko, Hatzenbuehler, & Keyes, 2014). These data exist within the larger context of the Trump administration threatening to repeal parts of the Affordable Care Act, including protections for SGMs which would further compound existing heart, brain, and mental health disparities (Williams & Anderson, 2020). The following examples highlight the disproportionate impact of structural stigma on specific racial/ethnic LGBTQ groups; this level of analysis may be a good starting point to inform interventions using policy in the United States and other countries around the globe.

HIV and Black and Latinx Men

As a chronic health condition, the Human Immunodeficiency Virus (HIV) disproportionately affects Black and Latinx men who have sex with men (MSM), who often experience higher rate of HIV-related societal stigma (CDC, 2020). HIV-related societal stigma refers to negative attitudes toward people living with HIV (PLWH). This stigma is associated with detrimental health behaviors such as lower medication adherence, less contact with medical providers, and increased risk of substance use (Sayles, Wong, Kinsler, Martins, & Cunningham, 2009). Moreover, policies that criminalize HIV contribute to this stigma. As of 2019, 34 states had laws that criminalize HIV exposure (Center for HIV Law and Policy [CHLP], 2020). These laws require PLWH to disclose their positive serostatus to prospective partners. Violations of such laws are treated as felonies, with convictions requiring sex offender registration. Yet, research suggests these laws do not significantly increase safer sex practices and they disproportionately affect Black MSM (Galletly, Pinkerton, & DiFranceisco, 2012). Additionally, these laws criminalize the sexual behavior of PLWH, which only further perpetuates societal stigma (CHLP, 2020). Besides affecting those who are PLWH, structural stigma contributes to lower rates of pre-exposure prophylaxis (PrEP) uptake and medication shown to prevent HIV, and it is associated with higher rates of risky sexual behavior among Black and Latinx MSM compared to white MSM (Buck, 2020).

Immigrants and Asylum Seekers

LGBTQ immigrants and asylum seekers are subjected to structural stigma. Until 1990, being a sexual minority was grounds for denial of immigration to the United States (Rank, 2002). LGBTQ people face persecution in many countries around the world, prompting many to flee to another country for safety (Itaborahy & Zhu, 2014). Moreover, 71% of undocumented LGBTQ immigrants are Latinx (Gates, 2013). In recent years, immigration and asylum laws have become increasingly restrictive, and extended detention of asylum seekers is commonplace in the United States. Detention centers often create and exacerbate mental health problems, and detainees are often at high risk for experiencing further violence from other detainees and even detention officers (APA, 2019). Recent evidence has highlighted these injustices, with some scholars finding that Latinx transgender asylum seekers who experience lengthy detentions are subjected to dehumanization, abuse, and transphobia in detention, including being denied access to basic human needs and medical care (Minero, 2020). This abuse is also associated with negative psychological health, including anxiety, depression, and suicidality (Minero, 2020).

Violence toward Transgender Women of Color

Transgender women of color (TWoC), especially Black and multiracial transwomen, experience poorer health and higher rates of morbidity, resulting from relative to sexual minority populations (Coursolle, 2019; James et al., 2016). TWoC are more likely to be homeless and engaged in sex work, leaving them increasingly vulnerable to additional health problems, like sexually transmitted infections (STIs), mental health diagnoses, and early death, compared to white transgender women (James et al., 2016; Jamosko, 2019). There are a number of legal defense policies that maintain and perpetuate further maltreatment against TWoC. For example, there is the continued use and support of the trans panic defense. Originally coined as the "gay panic defense," this legal defense is used to reduce the severity of a murder charge, particularly when the murderer is a cisgender and heterosexual white man and the victim is a TWoC, claiming that a perpetrator acted in self-defense against a victim (The National LGBT Bar Association, 2020). The problem with the use, and success, of this defense is that it is not only an injustice to the victim but also works to further perpetuate stereotypes of transgender individuals (Lee & Kwan, 2014). To this end, TWoC are often criminalized and have limited access to social support to help them survive and thrive. Among this already extremely marginalized group, it is vital to recognize that Black transgender women have high rates of health problems, homelessness, sex work, police brutality, and incarceration relative to white transwomen (Center for American Progress, 2016).

Sex Workers and Police Brutality

Given the high rates of job discrimination and lack of opportunities for higher education and necessary services to aid in employment, LGBTQ individuals, particularly TWoC, often engage in sex work as a means of income, support, and survival (Fitzgerald, Elspeth, Hickey, Biko, & Tobin, 2015). LGBTQ individuals, especially those who are homeless, are seven times more likely to trade sex for a place to stay (Fitzgerald et al., 2015). Black and Latinx gay men and transwomen are more likely than their white gay and transwomen counterparts to engage in sex work (Fitzgerald et al., 2015; James et al., 2016). This form of work can be very dangerous, as there is a high risk of STIs, assault, felony charges, and police brutality. In states where sex work is criminalized, there is a significant limit in access to health care, no safe and secure screening of clients, no labor rights for those who engage in this legitimate form of work, and hostile interactions between sex workers and police often occur (Fitzgerald et al., 2015). Indeed, transgender sex workers report a very high interaction with police (Fitzgerald et al., 2015). During these interactions, over 50% reported feeling uncomfortable and experience mistreatment by police in the form of verbal harassment, as well as physical and sexual assault. On average, TWoC, especially Black and multiracial transwomen, are more than twice as likely than white transgender persons to get arrested for crimes related to being transgender; there is an even higher arrest rate for "any reason whatsoever" (Center for American Progress, 2016; Fitzgerald et al., 2015). Additionally, transgender PoC often receive harsher charges, as well as increased hostile interactions, in which police often confiscate or destroy the condoms they use to protect themselves compared to white transwomen (Center for American Progress, 2016; Fitzgerald et al., 2015). Furthermore, TWoC who are sex workers are also homeless (Center for American Progress, 2016; Fitzgerald et al., 2015). Along with daily instances of discrimination, TWoC also experience lawful discrimination when seeking aid from homeless shelters, and Black transwomen are significantly more likely to be turned away than white transwomen and other TWoC (Barr, 2020; Fitzgerald et al., 2015). Thus, these policies limit access to resources, create hostile environments for sex workers, particularly TWoC, and further stigmatize and shape society's view of these communities, all of which have a negative impact on TWoC health.

Incarcerated LGBTQ PoC

LGBTQ PoC are overrepresented in the criminal justice system. For example, 85% of LGBTQ youth currently in the juvenile justice system are PoC (40% are African American youth), which is often the result of racial/ ethnic discrimination and profiling (Center for American Progress, 2016). Moreover, LGBTQ PoC are charged at higher rates than white LGBTQ individuals, leading to a disproportionate number of LGBTQ PoC in prisons (Center for American Progress, 2016). Not only are there more LGBTQ PoC incarcerated each year than white LGBTQ individuals, Black transgender women are incarcerated at a rate that is ten times that of the general population (Fitzgerald et al., 2015). Once incarcerated, LGBTQ PoC experience physical and sexual assault, increased use of solitary confinement, and significant instances of violence targeting TWoC, particularly Black and Latina transwomen (National Center for Transgender Equality, 2018). While legally incarcerated individuals must be provided with basic health needs, there are no standards or policies in place to ensure high-quality health care, resulting in suboptimal health care for these communities (National Center for Transgender Equality, 2018). In fact, laws such as "inmate exclusions" bar incarcerated individuals from receiving any outside form of health care, meaning they are given doctors that typically use outdated and non-evidence-based forms of practice, further contributing to the marginalization and health disparities experienced by incarcerated racial/ethnic LGBTQ (Fiscella, Beletsky, & Wakeman, 2017).

WHAT CAN BE DONE?

From a macro level, the lack of data collection on sexual orientation and gender identity furthers structural stigma by blatantly ignoring the existence of LGBTQ people. While the 2020 Census' allowance of the option to identify a same-sex relationship may be considered a small victory, the Trump administration has rolled back much of the progress that was made on LGBTQ data collection under the Obama administration (National Center for Transgender Equality, 2020). For example, the Department of Health and Human Services removed demographic questions on sexual orientation and gender identity on national dataset and reports related to services for older adults, people with disabilities, foster youth, and foster/adoptive parents and guardians. This is in the context of already existing limited access to health care, economic instability, and unsupportive educational environments, all of which impact the health of racial/ethnic LGBTQ (National Academies of Science, Engineering, and Medicine, 2020). Addressing these issues is imperative to tackling LGBTQ PoC heart, brain, and mental health disparities.

Structural stigma has historically affected the health and well-being of LGBTQ PoC. Most of the literature highlighting this has focused on risk factor perspectives, that is, identifying risk factors that increase disease burden. What is missing is a focus on resilience or strengths-based perspectives. Indeed, qualitative research suggests community strengths, such as safety and support, interconnectedness and resource sharing, and advocacy and collective action, have the potential to enhance health and well-being for Black, multiracial, and Latinx LGBTQ PoC (Hudson & Romanelli, 2020). Moreover, the Fenway Institute (2019), in a report detailing how Black LGBTQ people face intersectional adversities, calls for systemic change of institutional cultures that negatively impact the health of black LGBTQ people so that resilience can be promoted.

Regarding changing systems, governmental funds must be allocated to new and existing community-based organizations (CBOs) that serve LGBTQ PoC. An example of such structural changes is the recently passed California Assembly Bill (AB 2218) Transgender Equity and Wellness Fund (California Legislative Information, 2020). This California bill will now allow the state health department to provide funds to CBOs to improve access to health care, secure housing, food, and other life necessities specifically aimed for transgender communities, many of whom are PoC. Therefore, continued advocacy is needed from LGBTQ PoC allies, and the local and state government, to supplement the relentless work being done within these communities by existing CBOs. To this end, LGBTQ PoC should be treated with dignity, protected from discrimination, and be able to access the resources they need to end the health disparities that structural stigma creates. Improving LGBTQ PoC health is a long, difficult journey; however, if the road itself is changed, health equity can arise for LGBTQ PoC.

REFERENCES

American Psychological Association (2019). LGBTQ asylum seekers: How clinicians can help. Retrieved from https://www.apa.org/pi/lgbt/resources/lgbtq-asylum-seekers.pdf

Barr, K. (2020, July 28). *HUD rules promote discrimination, undermine equality.* National Law Center on Homelessness and Poverty. Retrieved from https://nlchp.org/new-hud-rules/

Buck, C. R. (2020). *Associations among state-Level structural Stigma, prevalence of PrEP use, and sexual risk-taking behavior among men who have sex with men* (master's thesis). Retrieved from ProQuest Dissertations Publishing. (27956692).

California Legislative Information. (2020). AB-2218 *Transgender wellness and equity fund*. Retrieved from https://leginfo.legislature.ca.gov/faces/billTextClient.xhtml?bill_id=201920200AB2218

Center for American Progress and Movement Advancement Project. (2016). *Unjust: How the broken criminal justice system fails LGBT people of color.* Retrieved from https://www.lgbtmap.org/file/lgbt-criminal-justice-poc.pdf

Centers for Disease Control and Prevention. (2020). Estimated HIV incidence and prevalence in the United States, 2014–2018. *HIV Surveillance Supplemental Report* 25(1). http://www.cdc.gov/hiv/library/reports/hiv-surveillance.html. Published May 2020. Accessed [date].

Correro, A. N., II, & Nielson, K. A. (2020). A review of minority stress as a risk factor for cognitive decline in lesbian, gay, bisexual, and transgender (LGBT) elders. *Journal of Gay & Lesbian Mental Health, 24*(1), 2–19. https://doi.org/10.1080/19359705.2019.1644570

Coursolle, A. (2019). *Protections for LGBTQ people with behavioral health needs.* National Health Law Program. Retrieved from https://healthlaw.org/resource/protections-for-lgbtq-people-with-behavioral-health-needs/

158   A. PRESCOTT ET AL.

Fiscella, K., Beletsky, L., & Wakeman, S. E. (2017). The inmate exception and reform of correctional health care. *American Journal of Public Health, 107*(3), 384–385. https://doi.org/10.2105/AJPH.2016.30362

Fitzgerald, E., Elspeth, S., Hickey, D., Biko, C., & Tobin, H. J. (2015). *Meaningful work: Transgender experiences in the sex trade*. Washington, DC: National Center for Transgender Equality.

Flores, A.R., Mallory, C., & Conron, K.J. (2020). *The impact of Obergefell v. Hodges on the well-being of LGBT Adults*. Los Angeles, CA: UCLA Williams Institute. Retrieved from https://escholarship.org/content/qt06f58379/qt06f58379.pdf

Fredriksen-Goldsen, K., Kim, H. J., Barkan, S., Muraco, A., & Hoy-Ellis, C. P. (2013). "Health Disparities Among Lesbian, Gay, and Bisexual Older Adults: Results From a Population-Based Study." *American Journal of Public Health, 103*(10), 1802–1809.

Galletly, C. L., Pinkerton, S. D., & DiFranceisco, W. (2012). A quantitative study of Michigan's criminal HIV exposure law. *AIDS Care, 24*(2), 174–179. https://doi.org/10.1080/09540121.2011.603493

Gates, G. J. (2013). LGBT Parenting in the United States. *The Williams Institute*, 1–6. https://escholarship.org/uc/item/9xs6g8xx

Goldenberg, T., Reisner, S. L., Harper, G. W., Gamarel, K. E., & Stephenson, R. (2020). State policies and healthcare use among transgender people in the U.S. *American Journal of Preventive Medicine, 59*(2), 247–259. https://doi.org/10.1016/j.amepre.2020.01.030

Hatzenbuehler, M. L. (2014). Structural stigma and the health of lesbian, gay, and bisexual populations. *Current Directions in Psychological Science, 23*(2), 127–132. https://doi.org/10.1177/0963721414523775

Hatzenbuehler, M. L., Jun, H., Corliss, H. L., & Bryn Austin, S. (2015). Structural stigma and sexual orientation disparities in adolescent drug use. *Addictive Behaviors, 46*, 14–18. https://doi.org/10.1016/j.addbeh.2015.02.017

Hudson, K. D., & Romanelli, M. (2020). "We are powerful people": Health-promoting strengths of LGBTQ communities of color. *Qualitative Health Research, 30*(8), 1156–1170. https://doi.org/10.1177/1049732319837572

Hughto, J. M. W., Reisner, S. L., & Pachankis, J. E. (2015). Transgender stigma and health: A critical review of stigma determinants, mechanisms, and interventions. *Social Science & Medicine, 147*, 222–231. https://doi.org/10.1016/j.socscimed.2015.11.010

Human Rights Campaign. (2020a). A history of federal non-discrimination legislation (93rd–114th Congress). Retrieved from https://www.hrc.org/resources/a-history-of-federal-non-discrimination-legislation

Human Rights Campaign. (2020b). Violence against the transgender community in 2020. Retrieved from https://www.hrc.org/resources/violence-against-the-trans-and-gender-non-conforming-community-in-2020

Itaborahy, L. P., & Zhu, J. (2014). State-sponsored homophobia—A world survey of laws: Criminalisation, protection and recognition of same-sex love. Retrieved from http://old.ilga.org/Statehomophobia/ILGA_SSHR_2014_ Eng.pdf

James, S. E., Herman, J. L., Rankin, S., Keisling, M., Mottet, L., & Anafi, M. (2016). *The report of the 2015 U.S. Transgender survey.* Washington, DC: National Center for Transgender Equality. Retrieved from https://www.transequality. org/sites/default/files/docs/usts/USTS%20Full%20Report%20-%20 FINAL%201.6.17.pdf

Jamosko, J. (2019). *Demographic data project: Gender minorities* [Scholarly project]. Retrieved from https://endhomelessness.org/wp-content/uploads/ 2019/06/Gender-Minority-Homelessness-Article-Revised-6-24-19- JJ-002.pdf

Lee, C., & Kwan, P. K. (2014). The trans panic defense: Heteronormativity, and the murder of transgender women. *Hastings Law Journal, 66*(1), 77–132. https://doi.org/10.2139/ssrn.2430390

Lukachko, A., Hatzenbuehler, M. L., & Keyes, K. M. (2014). Structural racism and myocardial infarction in the United States. *Social Science & Medicine, 103,* 42–50. https://doi.org/10.1016/j.socscimed.2013.07.021

Minero, L.P. (2020). *The impact of detention proceedings and solitary confinement on Latinx, transgender, undocumented and asylum seeking immigrants.* Retrieved from ProQuest Dissertations & Theses Global. (29028900).

National Academies of Sciences, Engineering, and Medicine. (2020). *Understanding the well-being of LGBTQI+ populations.* Washington, DC: The National Academies Press. https://doi.org/10.17226/25877.

National Center for Transgender Equality. (2018). *LGBTQ people behind bars: A guide to understanding the issues facing transgender prisoners and their legal rights.* Retrieved from https://transequality.org/sites/default/files/docs/ resources/TransgenderPeopleBehindBars.pdf

National Center for Transgender Equality. (2020). *The discrimination administration: Trump's record of action against transgender people.* Retrieved from https://transequality.org/the-discrimination-administration

National LGBT Health Education Center: A Program of the Fenway Institute. (2019). *Understanding and addressing the social determinants of health for Black LGBTQ people: A way forward for health centers.* Retrieved from https:// www.lgbtqiahealtheducation.org/wp-content/uploads/2019/06/TFIE-33_ SDOHForBlackLGBTPeople_Web.pdf

Pachankis, J. E., Hatzenbuehler, M. L., & Starks, T. J. (2014). The influence of structural stigma and rejection sensitivity on young sexual minority men's daily tobacco and alcohol use. *Social Science & Medicine, 103,* 67–75. https://doi. org/10.1016/j.socscimed.2013.10.005

Perez-Brumer, A., Hatzenbuehler, M. L., Oldenburg, C. E., & Bockting, W. (2015). Individual- and structural-level risk factors for suicide attempts among transgender adults. *Behavioral Medicine, 41*(3), 164–171. https://doi. org/10.1080/08964289.2015.1028322

Rank, L. (2002). Gays and lesbians in the U.S. immigration process. *Peace Review, 14*, 373–377. https://doi.org/10.1080/1040265022000039141

Sayles, J. N., Wong, M. D., Kinsler, J. J., Martins, D., & Cunningham, W. E. (2009). The association of stigma with self-reported access to medical care and antiretroviral therapy adherence in persons living with HIV/AIDS. *Journal of General Internal Medicine, 24*(10), 1101–1108. https://doi.org/10.1007/s11606-009-1068-8

The Center for HIV Law and Policy. (2020). *HIV criminalization in the United States: A sourcebook on state and federal HIV criminal law and practice.* Retrieved from http://www.hivlawandpolicy.org/sourcebook

The National LGBT Bar Association. (2020). *LGBTQ+ "panic" defense.* Retrieved from https://lgbtbar.org/programs/advocacy/gay-trans-panic-defense/

U.S. Department of Veteran Affairs. (2020). *Veterans with lesbian, gay, bisexual and transgender (LGBT) and related identities.* Retrieved from https://www.patientcare.va.gov/LGBT/index.asp

Wight, R. G., LeBlanc, A. J., & Badgett, M. V. L. (2013). Same-sex legal marriage and psychological well-being: Findings from the California Health Interview Survey. *American Journal of Public Health, 103*(2), 339–346. https://doi.org/10.2105/AJPH.2012.301113

Williams, N.D., & Anderson, E.A. (2020). A critique of repealing the Affordable Care Act: Implications for queer people of color. *Analyses of Social Issues and Public Policy.* https://doi.org/10.1111/asap.12197.

CHAPTER 13

Future Directions: Using Current Knowledge to Inform the Future of LGBTQ PoC Heart, Brain, and Mental Health Disparities

James J. García

Abstract LGBTQ PoC continue to face oppression in the U.S. and across the globe. This chapter highlights how this oppression, as unique minority stress in the form of intersectional discrimination, impacts the heart, brain, and mental health of racial/ethnic LGBTQ by summarizing key findings from each chapter to inform the future directions of research, practice, and advocacy of LGBTQ PoC health. The chapter also makes some methodological considerations related to the study of racial/ethnic LGBTQ health. Attention is paid to standardization of the assessment of race/ethnicity, sexual orientation/gender identity, and stresses that major PoC datasets should contain LGBTQ PoC persons in order to facilitate comparisons and highlight health disparities for racial/ethnic LGBTQ.

J. J. García (✉)
Department of Psychology, School of Health and Community Well-Being,
University of La Verne, La Verne, CA, USA
e-mail: JGarcia4@laverne.edu

J. J. García (ed.), *Heart, Brain and Mental Health Disparities for
LGBTQ People of Color*,
https://doi.org/10.1007/978-3-030-70060-7_13

161

Keywords Intersectional Discrimination • Resilience • LGBTQ older adults

LGBTQ PoC continue to face oppression in the U.S. and across the globe. This edited collection highlights how this oppression, as unique minority stress in the form of intersectional discrimination, impacts the heart, brain, and mental health of racial/ethnic LGBTQ. This chapter will provide highlights from each chapter to inform the future directions of research, practice, and advocacy to promote the heart, brain, and mental health of LGBTQ PoC.

The first four chapters of this edited text provide strong theoretical rationale for three key frameworks. For example, Chap. 2 introduces the concept of minority stress and focuses on intersectional discrimination (ID) as a specific type of stress that racial/ethnic LGBTQ experience in societies. The authors stress that ID results in chronic and sustained activation of the stress response, which then leads to psychosocial battle fatigue for many sexual and gender minority persons of color (SGMoC) (Ramirez & Paz Galupo, 2019). Moreover, Chap. 3 goes into detail on why the perspective of intersectionality is important to center in LGBTQ PoC health. In particular, this chapter explains that it is not identities that are inherently a risk for adverse health; rather it is the social stigma and marginalization directed toward people with intersectional identities that create hostile and toxic interactions that harm LGBTQ PoC health (Carbado, Crenshaw, Mays, & Tomlinson, 2013). Importantly, it is naïve to tease apart identities, as a means to reduce them to isolated components, as people do not exist in this manner—the totality and social context under which our identities exist matters (Bowleg, 2013). Chapter 4 provides a physiological framework to understand the effects of intersectional discrimination as chronic and sustained wear and tear of the body for LGBTQ PoC. Specifically, the allostatic load burden of LGBTQ PoC is highlighted in order to understand that the unique stressors have real health consequences for racial/ethnic LGBTQ people—namely the heart, brain, and mental health for these communities (Parra & Hastings, 2018).

As the first in the heart health section, Chap. 5 highlights the importance of examining cardiovascular disease (CVD) burden for LGBTQ PoC. In particular, there are specific areas of growth to further understand heart health, including the need for longitudinal research designs, using objective measures of CVD burden (e.g., physiologically based biomarkers), using existing frameworks like the American Heart Association's (AHA's) Life's Simple 7 as standardized cardiovascular metrics with LGBTQ PoC (Caceres et al., 2020), and using separate statistical analyses to examine differences for racial/ethnic LGBTQ. Chapter 6 focuses on the comorbidity of CVDs and human immunodeficiency virus (HIV), but indicates there are few studies focused on the unique associations of intersectional discrimination that examine both CVDs and HIV as comorbid disorders (Rich et al., 2020). Additionally, a focus on LGBTQ PoC living without HIV and who have high CVD risk factor (RF) burden is largely missing to inform prevention strategies for these communities.

The second section introduces brain health, focusing on stroke and the impact of HIV on the brain of LGBTQ PoC. Chapter 7 provides compelling evidence that there is high stroke RF burden for SGMoC, but also highlights several areas that are underexplored in the literature. In particular, there is a lack of objective indicators used to quantify stroke burden, limited data on stroke prevalence outside of the context of comorbid HIV, minimal data on the associations of ID on stroke risk, and no differentiation of stroke type. Moreover, current studies do not mirror national initiatives, like Life's Simple 7, to promote comparability between larger national sample datasets and those from studies with LGBTQ PoC. There are also no data on the impact of psychosocial factors, like intersectional discrimination, within the inpatient rehabilitation continuum of care for LGBTQ PoC; this is an untested but plausible hypothesis, as there are emerging data indicating that racial/ethnic discrimination plays a role in poststroke inpatient rehabilitation functioning for PoC (García & Warren, 2019). Current studies also do not examine the calibrated models often used to predict future stroke risk with LGBTQ PoC populations, though some research has examined Framingham Risk Scores in lesbian and bisexual women (Farmer, Jabson, Bucholz, & Bowen, 2013). Chapter 8 continues the focus on brain health but in the context of HIV. This chapter proposes that although highly active antiretroviral therapy (HAART) is a game changer, neurocognitive impairments are evident for people living with HIV (PLWH) and it is plausible that LGBTQ PoC brain health is disproportionately affected by HIV; however, there are no studies focused on documenting or highlighting the prevalence of how HIV impacts the brain health of racial/ethnic LGBTQ. Moreover, neurocognition in LGBTQ older adults of color living with HIV is needed, given the invisibility of racial/ethnic LGBTQ older adults in the literature (van Sluytman & Torres, 2014).

Section three documents mental health disparities and highlights the risk and resilience perspectives for racial/ethnic LGBTQ. Chapter 9 centers the literature on ID that is associated with worse adverse mental health and higher risk for substance use—above and beyond experiencing marginalization in one identity—for LGBTQ PoC; however, a disaggregation of race/ethnicity must be done. Importantly, adolescence is a key period in the development of mental health disparities for LGBTQ PoC, but limited data exist on differences by race/ethnicity. Moreover, Chap. 10 describes the dominating risk perspective in the mental health disparities literature for LGBTQ PoC, with ID as a unique psychosocial stressor that increases risk of adverse mental health for these communities. Critically, the role of psychological mediators, as those posited within the psychological mediation framework (Hatzenbuehler, Nolen-Hoeksema, & Dovidio, 2009) is discussed and some key mediators of minority stress and psychological distress are identified for LGBTQ PoC (Ouch & Moradi, 2019). Systemic factors are highlighted to show that job insecurity, sex work, and access to health care are all important and impact mental health risk for LGBTQ PoC. As an alternative to the risk perspective, the authors highlight the need to focus on resilience in LGBTQ PoC, namely pride, spirituality/hope, community support, collective action, role models of resilience, civic engagement, and social justice action that allow SGMoC to resist discrimination. Moving forward, there is much need to empirical test pathways of resilience in heart, brain, and mental health outcomes for racial/ethnic LGBTQ persons (Perrin, Sutter, Trujillo, Henry, & Pugh Jr, 2020).

In the concluding chapters, critical attention is paid to the conceptualization of resilience for LGBTQ PoC and the role of structural stigma in the outcomes for these communities. In particular, Chap. 11 focuses on how resilience can be conceptualized in different ways and these have all received strong empirical support. A distinction between individual and community-level resilience sheds light on differences in the resilience experience of LGBTQ PoC, with intersectionality playing a role in this. In particular, the notion of syndemics is introduced to account for different experiences of resilience for LGBTQ PoC. Moreover, a focus on religiosity/spirituality for racial/ethnic LGBTQ is important, yet understudied. Regarding structural stigma, the authors argue in Chap. 12 that though we know much about this phenomenon with LGBTQ, limited attention has been paid to examining the effects of structural stigma with LGBTQ PoC in the context of heart, HIV, immigration, violence, sex work, police brutality, and incarcerated/justice-involved people. Importantly, the chapter focuses on highlighting how advocacy is important to promote LGBTQ PoC health, namely changing systems to provide health equity (versus equality). Examples of such efforts include legislation passed in California that earmarks state funds for community-based organizations that provide services addressing and promoting transgender wellness (California Legislative Information, 2020).

INFORMING THE FUTURE OF LGBTQ HEART, BRAIN, AND MENTAL HEALTH DISPARITIES RESEARCH

It seems daunting to take everything that impacts LGBTQ health and reduce it to several key future directions. Indeed, this practice perpetuates society's strong desire and need to simplify/reduce people's experiences, like using a cookbook recipe. This is an especially harmful practice to use when working with communities who have historically been marginalized and minoritized in societies. Instead, it is important to recognize that the health of LGBTQ PoC is affected, mediated, and impacted by individual and systemic factors, all of which contain unique experiences of intersectional discrimination, that increase risk. However, the narrative of racial/ethnic LGBTQ as all risk is only half of the story, as these communities also have rich narratives that highlight how they survive, thrive, and are resilient in their existence within societies.

That said, some key methodological suggestions can be made. First, assessment of sexual orientation and gender identities (SOGI) should be standardized in order to facilitate comparison of data collection between datasets. To this end, the Williams Institute at the University of California at Los Angeles has developed guidelines to inform the assessment of SOGI (Williams Institute, 2019). Moreover, it is also essential for capturing race/ethnicity data, as there must be standardization in the assessment of this variable to compare across different heart, brain, and mental health datasets. One way to standardize the collection of race/ethnicity is to use governmental standards for collecting race and ethnicity; though outdated, guidance from the Office of Management and Budget's (OMB, 1997) directive remains the most widely used way to assess race/ethnicity. Second, a focus on research using objective indicators of disease burden is important in order to document the physiological toll of minority stress, in the form of intersectional discrimination, for LGBTQ PoC. Similar to large-scale epidemiological studies solely focused on LGBTQ like the 2014 federally funded National Health, Aging, and Sexuality/Gender Study, Aging with Pride (Fredriksen-Goldsen & Kim, 2017), the 2006 National Heart, Lung, and Blood Institute's Hispanic/Latinx people (Hispanic Community Health Study/Study of Latinos [HCHS/SOL]; Sorlie et al., 2010),the National Institutes of Health subclinical heart disease in South Asians (Mediators of Atherosclerosis in South Asians Living in America [MASALA]; Kanaya et al., 2013), and the population-based longitudinal racial/ethnic differences in stroke (Reasons for Geographic and Racial Differences in Stroke [REGARDS]; Howard et al., 2005), there is a need to create such a study to systematically examine heart, brain, and mental health exclusively in racial/ethnic LGBTQ samples. Importantly, the centering of intersectional discrimination is vital to accurately capture the heart, brain, and mental health of racial/ethnic LGBTQ (Cyrus, 2017). Moreover, there must be deliberate efforts to recruit and respectfully study the experiences of transgender and gender diverse persons, as current studies examine health disparities in trans persons by examining their similar biological sex heterosexual counterparts (i.e., trans man is compared to a cisgender woman), which does not respect the trans or gender diverse identity of the person. Additionally, this text was written and published during the worst pandemic in history (COVID-19) and there are few efforts focused on the heart and brain of racial/ethnic LGBTQ; this edited text would be remissed if it did not mention that health disparities during COVID-19 disproportionately impacted LGBTQ PoC. Together, the inclusion of some of these suggestions can facilitate comparisons with national datasets, in order to highlight differences in health and health disparities for SGMoC compared to other populations. Incorporating these methodological suggestions will center the unique health risks, resilience, and unmet needs for these communities of LGBTQ PoC in the U.S. and across the globe.

REFERENCES

Bowleg, L. (2013). "Once you've blended the cake, you can't take the parts back to the main ingredients": Black gay and bisexual men's descriptions and experiences of intersectionality. Sex Roles, 68(11–12), 754–767. https://doi.org/10.1007/s11199-012-0152-4

Caceres, B. A., Streed, C. G. Jr, Corliss, H. L., Lloyd-Jones, D. M., Matthews, P. A., Mukherjee, M., ... American Heart Association Council on Cardiovascular and Stroke Nursing; Council on Hypertension; Council on Lifestyle and Cardiometabolic Health; Council on Peripheral Vascular Disease; and Stroke Council. (2020). Assessing and addressing cardiovascular health in LGBTQ adults: A scientific statement from the American Heart Association. *Circulation, 142,* e1–e12. https://doi.org/10.1161/CIR.0000000000000914

California Legislative Information. (2020). AB-2218 Transgender wellness and equity fund. Retrieved from https://leginfo.legislature.ca.gov/faces/billText-Client.xhtml?bill_id=201920200AB2218

Carbado, D. W., Crenshaw, K. W., Mays, V. M., & Tomlinson, B. (2013). Intersectionality: Mapping the movements of a theory. *Du Bois Review: Social Science Research on Race, 10*(2), 303–312. https://doi.org/10.1017/S1742058X13000349

Cyrus, K. (2017). Multiple minorities as multiply marginalized: Applying the minority stress theory to LGBTQ people of color. *Journal of Gay & Lesbian Mental Health, 21*(3), 194–202. https://doi.org/10.1080/1935970 5.2017.1320739

Farmer, G. W., Jabson, J. M., Bucholz, K. K., & Bowen, D. J. (2013). A population-based study of cardiovascular disease risk in sexual-minority women. *American Journal of Public Health, 103*(10), 1845–1850. https://doi.org/10.2105/AJPH.2013.301258

Fredriksen-Goldsen, K. I., & Kim, H. J. (2017). The science of conducting research with LGBT older adults-an introduction to aging with pride: National Health, aging, and sexuality/gender study (NHAS). *The Gerontologist, 57*(suppl_1,1), s1–s14. https://doi.org/10.1093/geront/gnw212

García, J. J., & Warren, K. L. (2019). Race/ethnicity matters: Differences in Poststroke inpatient rehabilitation outcomes. *Ethnicity & Disease, 29*(4), 599–608. https://doi.org/10.18865/ed.29.4.599

Hatzenbuehler, M. L., Nolen-Hoeksema, S., & Dovidio, J. (2009). How does stigma "get under the skin?": The mediating role of emotion regulation. *Psychological Science, 20*(10), 1282–1289. https://doi.org/10.1111/j.1467-9280.2009.02441.x

Howard, V. J., Cushman, M., Pulley, L., Gomez, C. R., Go, R. C., Prineas, R. J., ... Howard, G. (2005). The reasons for geographic and racial differences in stroke study: Objectives and design. *Neuroepidemiology, 25*(3), 135–143. https://doi.org/10.1159/000086678

Kanaya, A. M., Kandula, N., Herrington, D., Budoff, M. J., Hulley, S., Vittinghoff, E., & Liu, K. (2013). Mediators of atherosclerosis in south Asians living in America (MASALA) study: Objectives, methods, and cohort description. *Clinical Cardiology, 36*(12), 713–720. https://doi.org/10.1002/clc.22219

Office of Management and Budget. (1997). Revisions to the standards for the classification of federal data on race and ethnicity. Retrieved from https://www.whitehouse.gov/wp-content/uploads/2017/11/Revisions-to-the-

Standards-for-the-Classification-of-Federal-Data-on-Race-and-Ethnicity-October30-1997.pdf

Ouch, S., & Moradi, B. (2019). Cognitive and affective expectation of stigma, coping efficacy, and psychological distress among sexual minority people of color. *Journal of Counseling Psychology, 66*(4), 424–436. https://doi.org/10.1037/cou0000360

Parra, L. A., & Hastings, P. D. (2018). Integrating the neurobiology of minority stress with an intersectionality framework for LGBTQ-Latinx populations. *New Directions for Child and Adolescent Development, 161*, 91–108. https://doi.org/10.1002/cad.20244

Perrin, P. B., Sutter, M. E., Trujillo, M. A., Henry, R. S., & Pugh, M., Jr. (2020). The minority strengths model: Development and initial path analytic validation in racially/ethnically diverse LGBTQ individuals. *Journal of Clinical Psychology, 76*(1), 118–136. https://doi.org/10.1002/jclp.22850

Ramirez, J. L., & Paz Galupo, M. (2019). Multiple minority stress: The role of proximal and distal stress on mental health outcomes among lesbian, gay, and bisexual people of color. *Journal of Gay & Lesbian Mental Health, 23*(2), 145–167. https://doi.org/10.1080/19359705.2019.1568946

Rich, A. J., Williams, J., Malik, M., Wirtz, A., Reisner, S., DuBois, ... & Poteat, T. (2020). Biopsychosocial mechanisms linking gender minority stress to HIV comorbidities among black and Latina transgender women (LITE plus): Protocol for a mixed methods longitudinal study. *JMIR Research Protocols, 9*(4), e17076. https://doi.org/10.2196/17076

Sorlie, P. D., Avilés-Santa, L. M., Wassertheil-Smoller, S., Kaplan, R. C., Daviglus, M. L., Giachello, A. L., ... LaVange, L. (2010). Design and implementation of the Hispanic community health study/study of Latinos. *Annals of Epidemiology, 20*(8), 629–641. https://doi.org/10.1016/j.annepidem.2010.03.015

van Sluytman, L. G., & Torres, D. (2014). Hidden or uninvited? A content analysis of elder LGBT of color literature in gerontology. *Journal of Gerontological Social Work, 57*(2–4), 130–160. https://doi.org/10.1080/01634372.2013.877551

Williams Institute. (2019). UCLA School of Law Williams Institute LGBT data and demographics, LGBT proportion of Population: California. https://williamsinstitute.law.ucla.edu/visualization/lgbt-stats/?topic=LGBT&area=6#density

INDEX

A
Advocacy, 3
Allostatic load (AL), 6, 7, 20, 42–48,
    56, 62, 73, 74, 82, 84, 162
American Indians, 70
Asians, 19, 166

B
Bias, 18
Biphobia, 145
Black, 153
Brain, 2, 19, 20, 43, 82, 84, 94–100,
    129, 143, 145, 152,
    156, 162–166

D
Discrimination, 144
Disparities, 2, 4–6, 14–20, 45, 56, 60,
    62, 64, 82, 88, 110, 122–124,
    151–157, 162–166

H
Health behaviors, 57
Heart, 2, 4–7, 14, 19, 20, 42,
    44, 56, 61, 70, 71, 82, 88,
    129, 143, 145, 152,
    156, 162–166
Heterosexism, 98
HIV, 61
Homophobia, 111

I
Intersectional discrimination, 2,
    5–7, 17, 19, 20, 30, 31, 42,
    47–48, 56, 62–63, 72–75, 87,
    88, 98–99, 111–115, 124,
    125, 128, 141, 142, 144, 162,
    163, 165, 166
Intersectionality, 7, 16–18, 28–35, 42,
    57, 112, 116, 123–124, 138,
    141–142, 144, 145, 162, 164
Invisibility, 18